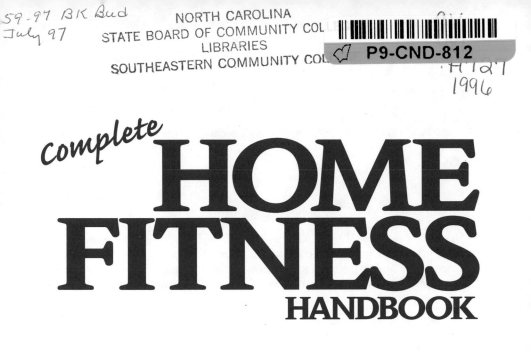

*Complete*

# HOME FITNESS HANDBOOK

### Edmund R. Burke, PhD
University of Colorado at Colorado Springs

Editor

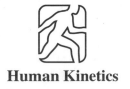

**Human Kinetics**

## Library of Congress Cataloging-in-Publication Data

Complete home fitness handbook / Edmund R. Burke, editor.
   p.  cm.
   ISBN 0-87322-994-0
   1.  Physical fitness.   2.  Exercise--Equipment and supplies.
  I.  Burke, Ed, 1949-  .
  GV481.H727   1996
  613.7'1--dc20                               95-38818

ISBN: 0-87322-994-0

Exercise and health are matters that vary from person to person. Readers should speak with their own doctors about their individual needs before starting any exercise program. This book is not intended as a substitute for the medical advice and supervision of your personal physician. Any application of the recommendations set forth in the following pages is at the reader's discretion and sole risk.

"Assessing Your Health" (pp. 13-16) from *Jog, Run, Race* (pp. 20-22), by Joe Henderson, 1978, Mountain View, CA: Anderson World. Copyright 1978 by Anderson World. Adapted with permission. Table 11.7 (p. 200) from *Nutrition, Weight Control, and Exercise, 4th Edition* (p. 227), by Frank Katch and William McArdle, 1993, Philadelphia: Lea & Febiger. Copyright 1993 by Katch and McArdle. Adapted with permission. Photos: p. 3 © Trek USA; p. 5 © Life Fitness; p. 8 © *Home Gym and Fitness* magazine; p. 27 © Photo Concepts/John Kilroy; p. 61 © Soloflex, Inc.; p. 62 © Trimax; p. 63 © Keiser Corporation; p. 184 © Will Zehr; pp. 223 and 226 © Chris Brown; p. 238 © Nautilus; p. 244 courtesy of Polar Electro, Inc.; All other photos © Schwinn Cycling & Fitness, Inc.

**Developmental Editor:** Julia Anderson; **Assistant Editor:** Jacqueline Eaton Blakley; **Editorial Assistant:** Coree Schutter; **Copyeditor:** Barbara Field; **Proofreader:** Dawn Barker; **Typesetting and Text Layout:** Ruby Zimmerman and Tara Welsch; **Text Designer:** Stuart Cartwright; **Photo Editor:** Boyd LaFoon; **Cover Designer:** Jack Davis; **Photographer (cover):** Dennis Lane; **Printer:** United Graphics

Printed in the United States of America    10  9  8  7  6  5  4  3  2  1

**Human Kinetics**
P.O. Box 5076, Champaign, IL 61825-5076
1-800-747-4457

*Canada*: Human Kinetics, Box 24040, Windsor, ON N8Y 4Y9
1-800-465-7301 (in Canada only)

*Europe:* Human Kinetics, P.O. Box IW14, Leeds LS16 6TR, United Kingdom
(44) 1132 781708

*Australia:* Human Kinetics, 2 Ingrid Street, Clapham 5062, South Australia
(08) 371 3755

*New Zealand:* Human Kinetics, P.O. Box 105-231, Auckland 1
(09) 523 3462

# Contents

# Foreword

As a young, elite-level endurance athlete, my long-term goals were to make the Olympics and win a medal. I was lucky to achieve both of these goals, competing in the Olympics twice and winning the gold at Munich in 1972.

When my Olympic days were over, I continued to train at nearly the same level of intensity, not primarily to compete, but because I found I enjoyed the training: It was part of my life. I felt better when I was in shape, and the stress release I experienced became more important than ever. I wanted to continue training for as long as possible, and when I could no longer run enough to satisfy my urge to exercise, I turned to other activities.

I have been cross-training for the past 12 years, using at least two of the training options featured in this book on a regular basis. Every individual, whether an athlete or a fitness enthusiast, should establish an exercise routine that involves endurance, strength, and flexibility training. Early in a fitness program, the primary emphasis can be aerobic, or endurance, training. Gradually, strength and flexibility will become more important. Clearly, when these fitness components are addressed, the quality—if not the length—of one's life can be increased.

If you try several different exercise routines and experiment with a few different pieces of home fitness equipment, you will find a mode of all-around exercise that suits you. Put in more technical terms, it's possible for everyone to discover a way of moving aerobically at an elevated heart rate that suits his or her unique biomechanical, physiological, and psychological endowments.

Over the years, because of time and family commitments, I've done more workouts in my home. But I still love to run outdoors. Running indoors on a treadmill is uncomfortable for me because I have spent so many years training and racing on the road and track. (I once averaged 17 miles a day over the course of a decade.) So instead of running, I ride a stationary bicycle. Why? Because, through trial and error, I have found that this particular apparatus suits me. My stair climber and cross-country ski machine are pleasant diversions, but I find more personal enjoyment on my stationary bike, which I can ride for 2 hours, 3 or 4 days in a row.

My body type (thin, ectomorphic) responds more reluctantly to weight training. The gains in both muscle mass and definition come slowly. Yet over the past 5 years, I have established an upper and lower body weight training routine on my multistation weight machine that has reversed subtle trends of the aging process.

As you age past 30, even if you are active, your muscles will start to atrophy. Even muscles you constantly use for vigorous activity will lose some of their mass unless you do some weight training. At the same time, your overall percentage of body fat will decrease. Today, at the age of 47, I am stronger than I was when I won the Olympic marathon at age 24, and my percentage of body fat has stabilized at what most would consider an enviable level. This is the result of year-round weight training, three to four times per week.

In addition to experimenting with various routines, I encourage you to be patient and follow your schedule for at least 2 months before passing judgment. Over the past 30 years of running and cross-training, I have come to the following conclusion: It takes the body approximately 2 weeks to adjust to any new physical activity. You have to get used to the movement and work your way through a period of awkwardness and some muscle soreness. Over the next 2 months, your body will adapt to the new activity. As it gets more comfortable at your level of exertion, you begin to feel in shape for that particular activity. Remember, 2 weeks to adjust, 2 months to adapt.

So experiment. Learn the training principles, and then try the home fitness exercise routines in this book. You're sure to enjoy the benefits of exercising without even having to step outside.

Good luck!
**Frank Shorter**

# chapter 1

# Finding Fitness at Home

**Edmund R. Burke, PhD**

*T*he three main reasons for the increased popularity of home fitness gyms and exercise are convenience, convenience, and convenience. For any fitness program to be successful, it must be done on a regular, sustained basis. With equipment in your home, you can roll out of bed, put on a pair of sweats, and start working out while the coffee is brewing.

For many, home workouts are easier to fit into their hectic schedules. No getting in the car and having to go to the health club. No standing in line to use the stair climber. Then there is the comfort and safety factor. Who wants to run outdoors during a raging blizzard, or to ride a bike on busy city streets during rush hour in the heat of summer? It's much more comfortable to hop on your stationary bicycle and exercise in the comfort and security of your air-conditioned home.

Privacy and cleanliness are also a big plus. Many feel intimidated in a gym, especially if they are carrying around a few extra pounds. At home you can exercise without feeling as though you are being rushed or that someone is pointing a finger at you. No more having to lie down on a sweaty bench or wondering if you'll catch athlete's foot in the shower.

But flexibility of time may be the biggest advantage. Today's demanding work and family schedules leave little room for flexibility. Parents with children soon discover that exercising at home turns out to be the only viable alternative if they want to stay fit. But parents and busy workers may not be the only ones who benefit from exercising at home.

# U.S. HEALTH CRISIS

Introducing regular exercise into your lifestyle is one of the smartest and most productive things you can do to maintain or improve your health. We know that 70 percent of all illnesses are lifestyle related. Over the last decade, many studies have reported convincingly that a long-term program of regular exercise and a proper diet can, in addition to preventing obesity, stave off a host of medical problems, including heart disease, diabetes, osteoporosis, and some forms of cancer.

In 1992, the American Heart Association (AHA) cited inactivity as a major contributing factor to heart disease. Following the lead of the AHA in 1993, the Centers for Disease Control and Prevention recommended that everyone in the country incorporate 30 minutes of physical activity into their daily lives.

And yet, less than 20 percent of all Americans are exercising on a regular basis. And half of those who start a program are no longer active 6 months later. Considering the benefits that exercise and a proper diet yield, why do so many have trouble starting and staying with an exercise program?

We're unprepared. Although many of us have the best intentions, we do not take the time to think through the process and formulate a plan. What kind of exercise do I like to do? Is my goal just to improve my health, or do I want to enter the local 10-kilometer run? We fail to ask simple questions or to give honest answers. However, if we do ask honest questions and set realistic goals, the results are going to point us down the right path.

# THE STANFORD HOME EXERCISE STUDY

In 1994, researchers at Stanford University School of Medicine conducted a year-long study of more than 350 subjects to examine the effectiveness and compliance of a group of supervised home exercisers versus individuals who reported for a group session at the university. The subjects were middle-aged men and women and included fit individuals as well as individuals who were overweight and smoked.

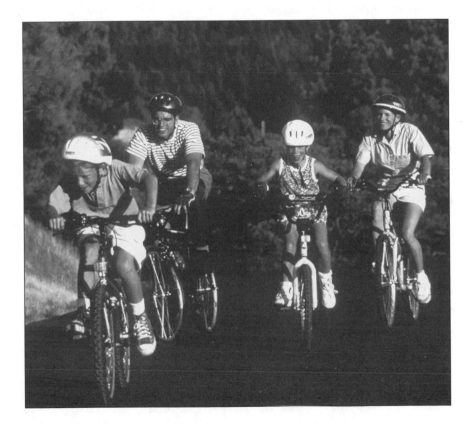

Exercisers in both the high-intensity (three 40-minute sessions per week on the treadmill at 73 to 88 percent of maximum heart rate, or MHR) and low-intensity (five 30-minute sessions at 60 to 71 percent of MHR) home exercise groups reported significantly greater adherence than those in the university-based program.

At the beginning of the study, many researchers predicted that the university-based group would have a greater compliance rate than the home-based group because of the camaraderie of the group and the instruction they received. But the study found the opposite to be true. The group program was just too inconvenient over the 12-month period for the subjects to justify the benefits.

The good news is that all three groups showed fitness improvements, with individuals in the low-intensity group achieving results similar to those in the high-intensity group. That should be strong motivation for those just starting a moderate exercise program.

Perhaps most importantly, research has also shown that it's never too late to start exercising . . . and experiencing the benefits. Studies conducted at Tufts University, for instance, show that even people in their 90s can significantly increase their strength as a result of following a moderate strength training program.

Exercise is one of life's joys. It energizes—giving you a sense of well-being and accomplishment and keeping you healthy and fit. There is great pleasure in being able to set goals, accept your own challenges, and push yourself to a better lifestyle of health and fitness.

# GETTING STARTED ON A FITNESS PROGRAM

Once you have made the commitment to get started on a home fitness program, here are some suggestions you may want consider to help you get off on the right foot and stay motivated. Remember that any new habit is difficult to establish at first, but it can be done. Follow these steps and you'll be on your way to establishing and using your home fitness center for improved health and fitness. After reading this section, refer to the Home Fitness Planning Worksheet (p. 6) and fill in the blanks. Use this information as a planning guide to get started on the road to fitness. Enjoy the journey!

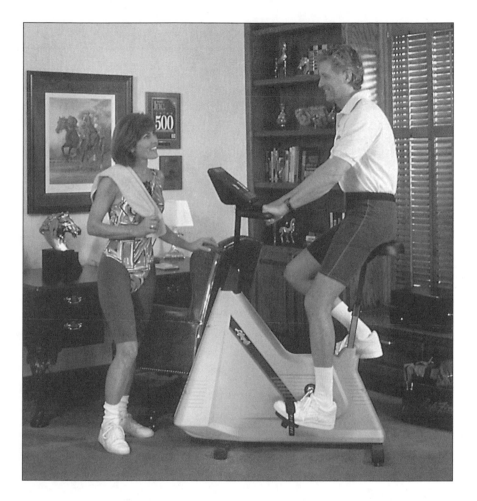

✔ Get a physical exam. If you have been inactive for several years or are new to an exercise program, be sure to consult with your family physician, especially if you're over 35, have health problems, or have a history of heart disease in your family.

✔ Begin planning for your home fitness center. Set aside a room or a portion of your house or apartment exclusively for fitness, and make sure that it's comfortable so you'll enjoy using it. If you enjoy music or like to look out a window while exercising, make sure these things are accessible. Don't force yourself to work out in a part of the house that isn't comfortable; you won't be motivated to exercise.

# HOME FITNESS PLANNING WORKSHEET

Target date to begin exercise program:_____

Times of day I can exercise:

    Time No. 1 _____

    Time No. 2 _____

    Time No. 3 _____

Days of the week that are good for me to work out:

    Day No. 1 _____

    Day No. 2 _____

    Day No. 3 _____

Activities I would like to experiment with:

    Activity No. 1 _____

    Activity No. 2 _____

    Activity No. 3 _____

Exercise goals I wish to accomplish:

    Goal No. 1 _____

    Goal No. 2 _____

    Goal No. 3 _____

Individuals who will support me in my exercise program:

    Person No. 1 _____

    Person No. 2 _____

    Person No. 3 _____

Individuals who can work out with me:

    Person No. 1 _____

    Person No. 2 _____

    Person No. 3 _____

✓ Do you need a companion? If you prefer to exercise with some-one, find a friend to train with who lives nearby. Encouraging your spouse or children to exercise with you is an excellent way to stay motivated and promote family unity.

✓ Determine what activities you like. Make a list of sports or activities that you currently enjoy the most or that you liked in your younger days. Choose sports that will add variety to your program, and vary your activities with the seasons.

✓ Find the right equipment. After you've decided what activities you like, start reviewing what home equipment is available to support those activities. Ask your friends who are into fitness or your local health club to recommend the names of reputable home fitness dealers. You'll find a much better selection of high-quality equipment and receive more professional service at a specialty store than at a discount or department store.

✓ Seek out good advice. If after reading this book you need addi-tional help in setting up a fitness program, contact a good health club. They offer many classes to help you get started or can recommend a personal trainer to work with you either at the club or at your home.

✓ Make fitness a part of your daily lifestyle. Include it in your daily planner, just as you would any other appointment. Keep the appointment; you'll be glad you did.

✓ Use affirmations. Positive affirmations will help you program your subconscious to accept new beliefs: I am living a healthier lifestyle by exercising several times a week at home. Repeat your affirmations several times each week.

The basics of any home fitness program are planning and setting goals. Goal setting and formulating a plan are the clearest ways of establishing a consistent program of exercise; they are also a power-ful form of direction and motivation. Take some time to think about what will help you begin your home exercise program and keep you motivated. Jot these ideas down on the Home Fitness Planning Worksheet. Don't spend time worrying about achieving these goals or about failing to exercise very many times a week in the beginning. However, do begin to imagine what kind of difference achieving your goals will have on your health, fitness, and overall appearance.

# DO YOU NEED A PERSONAL TRAINER?

If you lack motivation to work out at home, or just need someone to show you how to get the most out of your home equipment, a personal trainer might be the solution. Under the watchful eye of a trainer, many individuals sweat and strain to complete their workouts to the best of their abilities, especially when it's costing them $25 to $100 an hour.

You can find personal trainers in your area by looking through local newspapers and magazine ads and by asking for suggestions at your local health club or the place where you purchased your equipment. When shopping around for a personal trainer, interview several

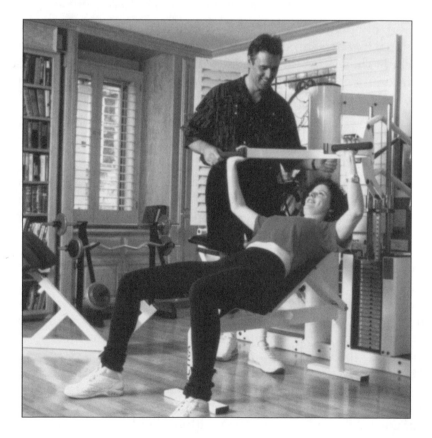

candidates carefully. Use the following questions during the initial interview.

Does the trainer have a background in exercise physiology, injury prevention, and monitoring exercise intensity, as evidenced by a degree or certification through a nationally recognized organization such as the National Strength and Conditioning Association (NSCA), the American Council on Exercise (ACE), or the American College of Sports Medicine (ACSM)? Does the trainer have experience in fitness training, and does he or she keep current with research through association membership, workshops, and journals?

Can the trainer design a program for you around your present home equipment? Does he or she recommend aerobic exercise, strength training, or a mixture of the two? Does the trainer know how to develop programs for nonaerobic sports such as volleyball, tennis, or golf?

Aerobic exercises are activities that require large amounts of oxygen for prolonged periods and will ultimately force your body to improve those systems responsible for the transportation of oxygen. These systems are often referred to as your cardiovascular system, because it is the heart and blood vessels that transport the oxygen to your working muscles. Examples of aerobic exercises are walking, jogging, lap swimming in a pool, a recreational bicycle ride, or cross-country ski touring.

Nonaerobic sports usually require short bursts of energy followed by periods of recovery. For example, in tennis, intense activity may take place for about 10 seconds, followed by a short period of recovery before the next serve. Some trainers refer to nonaerobic activities as power sports. Strength training usually requires lifting weight with a barbell, dumbbell, or a machine.

Is the trainer available when you want to work out? Does he or she have liability insurance? Does the trainer ask questions about your lifestyle? Does he or she help you set safe and realistic goals without promising unattainable results? Is the trainer willing to put in writing his or her workout methods? Are you comfortable with the trainer's gender?

The right chemistry must exist between trainer and trainee to get the most out of training. Eventually you'll come up with someone who can show you how to make the most of your exercise equipment and time.

# IT'S NEVER TOO LATE FOR FITNESS

Most of us have very busy schedules, and to keep our fitness intact we have to be extremely efficient. These three words, *efficiency of effort*, form the core of creating your own home fitness center. Efficiency of effort means producing maximum gains with minimal time spent, a goal most of us have when designing our home fitness programs.

The bottom line is that you must be creative and innovative to get the best results. With this book and your own creativity, a great workout is only a few moments away: a different grip on the multigym, a varied stepping rhythm on the stepper, a new intensity on the stationary wind-load simulator, or a more rapid stroke rate on the rower. By varying your workouts, you'll create maximum gains in the shortest time.

As you will see, your home fitness equipment will allow you to reach your fitness goals and prepare properly for a healthier lifestyle. Anyone who is serious about fitness—or for that matter, just wants to improve their overall fitness—should have a few basic pieces of home exercise equipment. It makes no difference whether you are a competitive cyclist or triathlete, or just someone trying to tone their muscles, the home fitness center is the most efficient way to help you reach your physical potential.

As you read this book, you should keep in mind that becoming knowledgeable about indoor training is only one of the essential ingredients in your personal recipe for sensible exercise. If you want to make your indoor exercise experience as productive and enjoyable as possible, you need to take several steps. The most crucial step is to make an unwavering commitment to exercise on a regular basis. For most individuals, that commitment will be based, at least in part, on understanding that regular aerobic exercise and strength training make sense for almost everyone and that exercise truly has medicinal properties.

You're in much better shape than most people—at least you've picked up a copy of this book! But you know you can get into even better shape, and that's why you're reading this book. Follow these guidelines and recommendations, and we know you'll come to realize the connection between balanced fitness and quality of life.

Explore this book. Read it in bits. And good luck as you begin using the equipment featured in this book in your balanced fitness program.

# chapter 2

# Checking Your Fitness

**Edmund R. Burke, PhD**

*B*efore you begin using the workout programs introduced in this book, we want you to take a few minutes to answer some questions about your current state of fitness and health. Many health benefits are associated with regular exercise. Completing this checklist is a sensible first step in increasing your physical activity. It will tell you whether you are ready for the home fitness self-test and with what level of training you may want to experiment. For many of us, physical activity poses no problem or hazard. Before you begin your home fitness program or other exercise requiring hard physical effort, we suggest you consult with your physician, particularly if you are over age 35, are overweight, smoke, or have a history of cardiovascular disease in your family.

## TESTING YOUR GENERAL HEALTH AND FITNESS

Before you begin the specific programs outlined in chapters 12 and 13, take a few minutes to answer the following questions. Afterward you will complete a fitness test, a compilation of four assessments to evaluate your current fitness level. These tests are not time-consuming and are easy to perform. You should enjoy the challenge, and the results will tell you much about your physical fitness.

Once you begin your home fitness program, you will want to test your improvement periodically. You will begin to feel better, but there is more to it. Numerous scientific studies show that you will see important physical changes over time. These changes are often hard to recognize because they occur gradually. That's why we recommend taking these tests about every 2 to 3 months. It will not only show your progress but will give you confidence that you are improving your health and fitness. As your score improves, you will enjoy a great sense of accomplishment and satisfaction.

# THE HOME FITNESS TEST

This test is the same for every adult, regardless of gender, age, or activity level; however, the results will differ according to those categories. These standards take these categories into account so that, for example, a 55-year-old male is not compared with a 45-year-old female.

Your results reflect acceptable standards for individuals in your age and gender group. But in the long run, you should only be comparing yourself to you. This will allow you to see clear improvements in fitness as your program progresses.

A highly fit individual will score more points for the four components than a low-fitness person, but many people will have varying scores. A good result in one category does not balance a poor score in another. Your ultimate goal is to score well in all categories after several months of training.

Table 2.1 describes the four components of the home fitness test. Each part has step-by-step instructions that are easy to follow and will help you perform the assessment properly. You may have to solicit the help of a family member or friend to ensure correct body positioning and confirm that you are doing each part of the test properly. You are now ready to begin your home fitness test.

| Table 2.1 | Fitness Test Components |
| --- | --- |

| Fitness Component | Assessment |
| --- | --- |
| Cardiovascular fitness | Rockport Walking Test (1 mi) |
| Muscular strength | Push-up or bench press test |
| Flexibility | Modified sit-and-reach test |
| Body composition | Body Mass Index |

## Assessing Your Health

### Cardiovascular Health:

Which of these statements best describes your cardiovascular condition? This is a critical safety check before you enter any vigorous activity. (Warning: If you have such a disease history, start the home exercise programs in this book only after receiving clearance from your doctor—and then only with close supervision by a personal trainer.)

No history of heart disease or circulatory problems ____(3)

Past ailments have been treated successfully ____(2)

Such problems exist but no treatment required ____(1)

Under medical care for cardiovascular disease ____(0)

### Injuries:

Which of these statements best describes your current injuries? This is a test of your musculoskeletal readiness to start a home fitness program. (Warning: If your injury is temporary, wait until it is cured before starting the program. If it is chronic, adjust the program to fit your limitations.)

No current injury problems ____(3)

Some pain in activity but not limited by the injury ____(2)

Level of activity is limited by the injury ____(1)

Unable to do much strenuous training ____(0)

*(continued)*

**Illnesses:**

Which of these statements best describes your current illnesses? Certain temporary or chronic conditions will delay or disrupt your exercise program. (See warning under previous section.)

No current illness problems _____(3)

Some problem with activity but not limited by it _____(2)

Level of activity is limited by the illness _____(1)

Unable to do much strenuous training _____(0)

**Age:**

Which of these age groups describes you? In general, the younger you are, the less time you have spent slipping out of shape.

Age 20 or younger _____(3)

Ages 21 to 29 _____(2)

Ages 30 to 39 _____(1)

Age 40 or older _____(0)

**Weight:**

Which of these figures describes how close you are to your own definition of ideal weight? Excess fat is a major indicator of unfitness, but it's also possible to be significantly underweight.

At or very near ideal body weight _____(3)

Less than 10 pounds above or below ideal weight _____(2)

10 to 19 pounds above or below ideal weight _____(1)

20 or more pounds above or below ideal weight _____(0)

**Resting Pulse Rate:**

Which of these figures describes your current pulse rate on waking up in the morning, before getting out of bed? A well-trained heart beats slower and more efficiently than one that's unfit.

Fewer than 60 beats per minute _____(3)

60 to 69 beats per minute _____(2)

70 to 79 beats per minute _____(1)

80 or more beats per minute _____(0)

## Smoking:

Which of these statements best describes your smoking habits and history (if any)? Smoking is the No. 1 enemy of health and fitness.

Never a smoker _____(3)

Once a smoker but quit _____(2)

An occasional, light smoker _____(1)

A regular, heavy smoker _____(0)

## Most Recent Exercise Outing:

Which of these statements best describes your exercise history within the last month? The best measure of how well you will be able to exercise at home in the near future is what recently took place in your exercise program.

Exercised nonstop for more than 1 hour _____(3)

Exercised nonstop for 30 minutes to 1 hour _____(2)

Exercised nonstop for less than 30 minutes _____(1)

No recent history of exercise _____(0)

## Exercise Background:

Which of these statements best describes your exercise history? Fitness does not last forever, but the fact that you were once involved in an organized fitness program at a health club or YMCA is a good sign that you will succeed at your new program.

Trained in an organized program within the
past year _____(3)

Trained in an organized program within the
past 1 or 2 years _____(2)

Trained in an organized program more than
2 years ago _____(1)

Never trained formally in an organized program _____(0)

*(continued)*

**Related Activities:**

Which of these statements best describes your participation in other sports and their overall aerobic and strength demands? The closer they relate to cycling, running, stair climbing (aerobic activities), and strength training, the better the carryover effect will be.

Regularly practice similar aerobic and
strength activities                                                    ____(3)

Regularly practice less vigorous aerobic
and strength activities                                                ____(2)

Regularly practice nonaerobic (bowling,
archery) and strength activities                                       ____(1)

Not regularly active in any physical activity                          ____(0)

Total Score:          _____

If you scored 20 points or more, you rate high in health and fitness for someone beginning or returning to a fitness program. You will probably progress rapidly in your fitness program.

Between 10 and 19 points, your score is average. You will need to begin the program slowly, and you will need to take a few days off every week.

A score of fewer than 10 points is below average. You will need to start slowly and may need the assistance of a personal trainer to help you get under way.

Adapted from Henderson (1978).

# TESTING CARDIOVASCULAR FITNESS

## ROCKPORT WALKING TEST

### Equipment:

A watch with a second hand or a stopwatch. If you own a heart rate monitor, use it to record your heart rate.

### Preparation:

1. Practice taking your pulse to determine your heart rate. This is not difficult, but it requires some practice. Your heart rate will be recorded in beats per minute. Using your index and middle fingers, locate your pulse at the base of your wrist or at the side of your neck near your Adam's apple (see Figure 2.1).

2. Do not eat, smoke, or drink coffee or tea for at least two hours before the test. In addition, don't participate in vigorous activity the previous day.

3. Wear loose-fitting clothing that allows you to exercise comfortably. Your shoes should be suited for walking.

4. Find a running track or a 1-mile flat loop:

   - A neighborhood school or college track
   - A YMCA or YWCA
   - A community fitness center or health club
   - A sidewalk along a flat street (measure in your car beforehand)

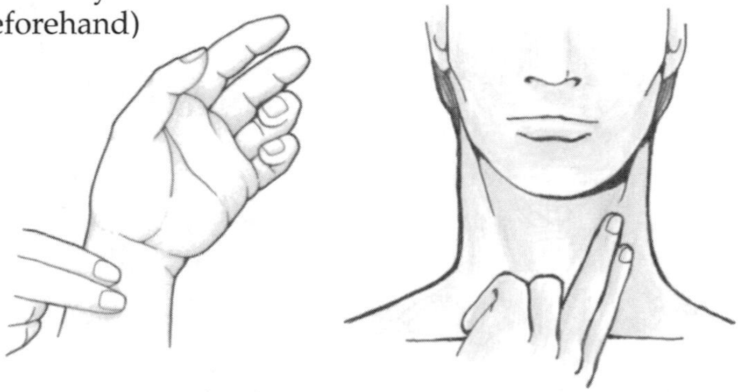

Figure 2.1 Locate your pulse to determine your heart rate.

## Procedure:

1. Warm up thoroughly. You can start by walking slowly and gradually increasing your pace until you feel warm or begin to perspire. I recommend some of the stretches listed in chapter 4.

2. Note the time or start the stopwatch and begin walking.

3. Stop walking after one mile, check your watch, and record your time to the nearest minute: _____ minutes.

4. Immediately locate your pulse, take for 15-second count, and multiply by four (or observe your heart rate on your heart rate monitor as you finish). Record your heart rate in beats per minute.

## Results:

1. Select the fitness chart (Figure 2.2) that matches your age and gender.

2. Locate your 1-mile walking time on the horizontal axis and draw a line straight up from that.

3. On the vertical axis, locate your heart rate upon completing the test, and draw a horizontal line to meet the vertical line. That point determines your cardiovascular fitness level.

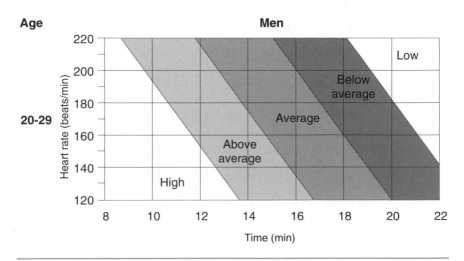

**Figure 2.2** Fitness charts for men and women at various ages.

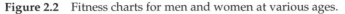

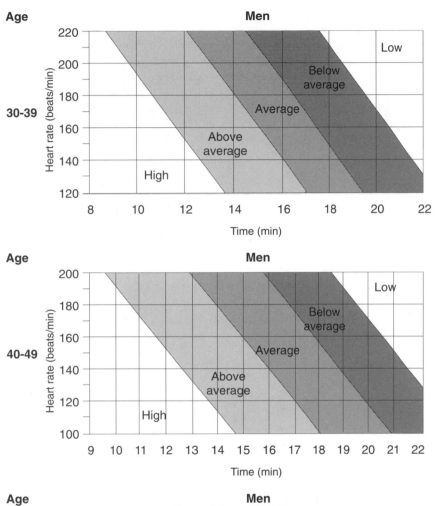

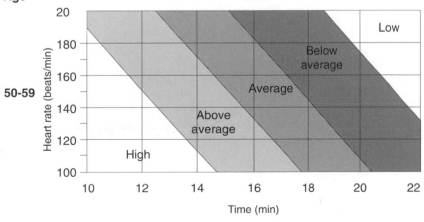

**Figure 2.2** *(continued)*

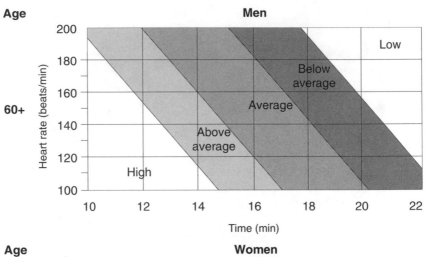

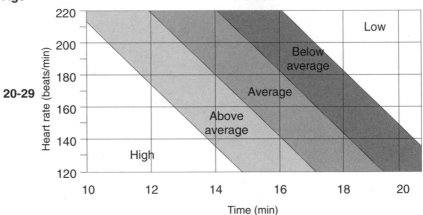

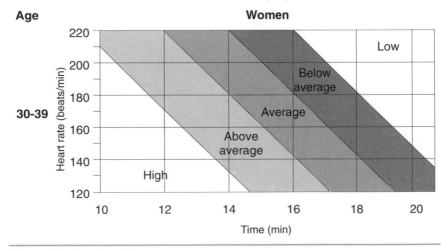

**Figure 2.2** *(continued)*

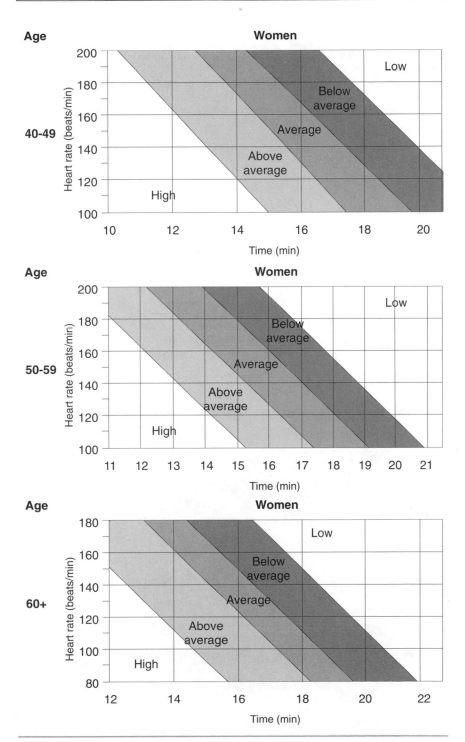

**Figure 2.2** *(continued)*

# EVALUATING MUSCULAR STRENGTH

Select either the push-up test or bench press test to test your muscular strength.

## PUSH-UP TEST

### Equipment:

None

### Preparation:

Warm up by performing some upper body stretches from chapter 4. Make sure you know how to perform a push-up correctly (men and women use different techniques, described here).

Position yourself on the floor so that your body is straight and your weight is on your hands and feet (men) or hands and knees (women). Be sure your hands are flat on the floor and directly under your shoulders .

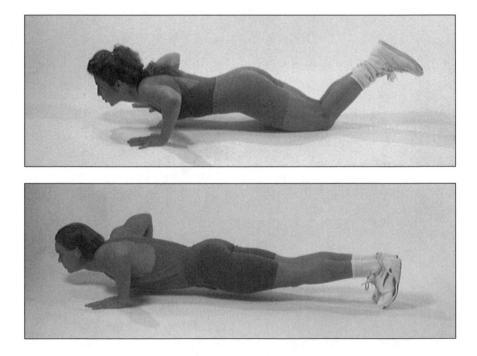

## Procedure:

1. Assume the correct position.
2. Begin the first push-up. Lower your chest until it touches the floor, then push yourself back up to the starting position. Exhale each time you push your body up; do not hold your breath. Keep your body straight, and fully straighten your arms at the end of each push-up.
3. Count each time you push up correctly.
4. Stop the test when you need to rest.
5. Record the number of push-ups you were able to do: _____.

## Results:

Compare your score to the standards in Table 2.2.

**Table 2.2   Muscular Fitness Norms (Push-Ups)**

| | Score at age | | | | |
|---|---|---|---|---|---|
| | 20-29 | 30-39 | 40-49 | 50-59 | 60+ |
| *Men* | | | | | |
| High | ≥ 45 | ≥ 35 | ≥30 | ≥ 25 | ≥ 20 |
| Average | 35-44 | 25-34 | 20-29 | 15-24 | 10-19 |
| Below average | 20-34 | 15-24 | 12-19 | 8-14 | 5-9 |
| Low | < 19 | < 14 | < 11 | < 7 | < 4 |
| *Women* | | | | | |
| High | ≥ 34 | ≥ 25 | ≥20 | ≥ 15 | ≥ 5 |
| Average | 17-33 | 12-24 | 8-19 | 6-14 | 3-4 |
| Below average | 6-16 | 4-11 | 3-7 | 1-5 | 1-2 |
| Low | < 5 | < 3 | < 2 | 0 | 0 |

From Pollock, Wilmore, and Fox, *Health and Fitness Through Physical Activity*. 1978. All rights reserved. Adapted by permission of Allyn & Bacon.

## BENCH PRESS TEST

If you have a free weight and bench or a multistation gym, this test will give you an idea of your general readiness to begin weight training.

### Equipment:

35-pound barbell for women
80-pound barbell for men
Flat bench (with uprights) or bench press station on multistation machine

### Procedure:

1. If you are using free weights, seek the help of a qualified individual to spot for you.

2. Lie on your back with your head, shoulders, upper back, and buttocks on the bench and your feet flat on the floor.

3. With your palms up, grip the bar at a position slightly wider than shoulder width.

4. With the spotter's assistance, move the bar upward and away from the uprights until your elbows are fully extended and the bar is directly above your nipples. Breathe out while pushing the weight.

5. Lower the bar to your chest while inhaling and pause.

6. Push the bar upward to a full elbow extension to complete the first repetition, and then return the bar to the chest and immediately press it again.

7. Continue pressing and lowering until you cannot complete another repetition. Perform each repetition in a slow and controlled manner. Allow 1 to 2 seconds for pushing the bar to the extended elbow position and 1 to 2 seconds for the downward movement to the chest. It should take 2 to 4 seconds to complete each repetition. Do not bounce the bar off your chest. As the repetitions become harder to complete, remember to breathe

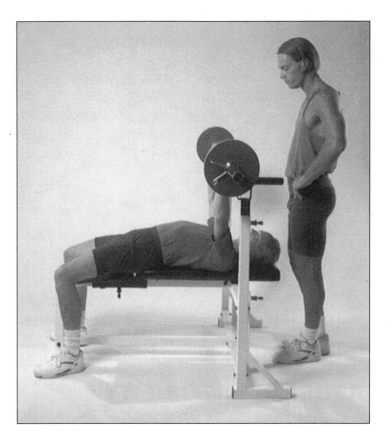

out when pushing upward and inhale during downward movements.

8. Record the number of repetitions you complete: _____.

## Results:

To determine your score, refer to the upper half of Table 2.3 if you are male and the lower half if you are female. Identify the appropriate age range column, and below it find the number of repetitions you completed. In the far left column, you'll find your weight training fitness level.

### Table 2.3 Muscular Fitness Norms (Bench Press)

**Fitness for weight training based on completed repetitions**

| Age | 18-25 | 26-35 | 36-45 | 46-55 | 56-65 | 66-75 |
|---|---|---|---|---|---|---|
| *Men* | | | | | | |
| High | ≥ 30 | ≥ 26 | ≥ 24 | ≥20 | ≥ 14 | ≥ 10 |
| Average | 21-29 | 18-25 | 15-23 | 10-19 | 7-13 | 5-9 |
| Low | ≤ 20 | ≤ 17 | ≤ 14 | ≤ 9 | ≤ 6 | ≤ 4 |
| *Women* | | | | | | |
| High | ≥ 28 | ≥ 25 | ≥ 21 | ≥ 20 | ≥ 16 | ≥ 12 |
| Average | 18-27 | 15-24 | 12-20 | 10-19 | 8-15 | 5-11 |
| Low | ≤ 17 | ≤ 14 | ≤ 11 | ≤ 9 | ≤ 7 | ≤ 4 |

Reprinted from Baechle and Earle (1995). Selected data from *Y's Way to Fitness* by J.A. Golding, C.R. Meyers, and W.E. Sinning, 1991, Chicago: National Board of YMCA.

# MEASURING FLEXIBILITY

## MODIFIED SIT-AND-REACH TEST

### Equipment:

Yardstick and adhesive tape

### Preparation:

1. Place the yardstick on the floor with the zero mark closest to you. Tape the yardstick in place at the 15-inch mark.

2. Ask a friend to help you keep your legs straight during the sit-and-reach test; however, it is important that he or she not interfere with your movement.

### Procedure:

1. Stretch properly using the exercises in chapter 4.

2. Sit on the floor with the yardstick between your legs, your feet 10 to 12 inches apart, and your heels even with the tape at the 15-inch mark.

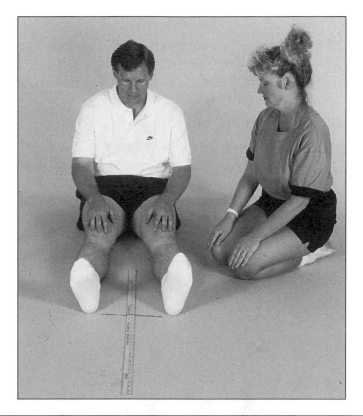

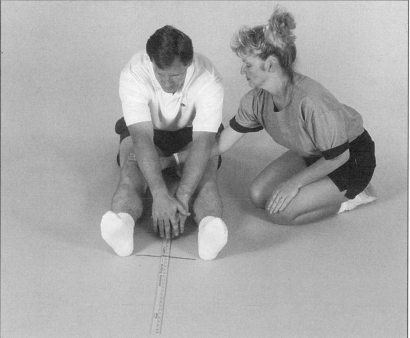

3. Place one hand over the other. The tips of your two middle fingers should be on top of one another.

4. Slowly stretch forward without bouncing or jerking and slide your fingertips along the yardstick as far as possible. The greater your reach, the higher your score will be.

5. Do the test three times.

6. Record your best score to the nearest inch: _____ inches.

## Results:

Compare your score to the standards in Table 2.4.

**Table 2.4   Modified Sit-and-Reach**

| | Score at age | | | | |
|---|---|---|---|---|---|
| | 20-29 | 30-39 | 40-49 | 50-59 | 60+ |
| *Men* | | | | | |
| High | ≥ 19 | ≥ 18 | ≥ 17 | ≥ 16 | ≥ 15 |
| Average | 13-18 | 12-17 | 11-16 | 10-15 | 9-14 |
| Below average | 10-12 | 9-11 | 8-10 | 7-9 | 6-8 |
| Low | < 9 | < 8 | < 7 | < 6 | < 5 |
| *Women* | | | | | |
| High | ≥ 22 | ≥ 21 | ≥ 20 | ≥ 19 | ≥ 18 |
| Average | 16-21 | 15-20 | 14-19 | 13-18 | 12-17 |
| Below average | 13-15 | 12-14 | 11-13 | 10-12 | 9-11 |
| Low | < 12 | < 11 | < 10 | < 9 | < 8 |

Reprinted from *ACSM Resource Manual for Guidelines for Exercise Testing and Prescription* (p. 165) by S. Blair, P. Painter, R.R. Pate, L.K. Smith, and C.B. Taylor, 1988, Philadelphia: Lea & Febiger, which was adapted from *The Y's Way to Physical Fitness* (pp. 106-111) by L.A. Golding, C.R. Myers, and W.E. Sinning (Eds.), 1982, Rosemont, IL: YMCA of the USA.

# ASSESSING BODY COMPOSITION

## BODY MASS INDEX

### Equipment:

Body Mass Index chart (Table 2.5), a body weight scale, and a ruler

### Preparation:

1. Wearing minimal clothing and no shoes, measure your body weight.

2. Measure your height; to get the most accurate measurement, remove your shoes, stand tall with heels together, and take a deep breath.

### Procedure:

1. On the Body Mass Index chart, locate your height (in inches) at the top of the scale.

2. Locate your weight (in pounds) on the left side of the scale.

3. Record the fitness category where the two values intersect: _____.

# THE FINAL SCORE

After completing the four parts of the home fitness test, it is time to review your results. Your four scores will give you a clear picture of your individual fitness profile, which will give you a basis upon which to gauge your improvements in fitness after you have been working out for a few weeks. We suggest that you retest yourself about every 2 to 3 months to monitor your progress and as a motivational tool to see that you are making gains in your overall fitness and health.

Now that you have a sense of your fitness level, we'll look at identification-specific fitness goals in the next chapter.

**Table 2.5  Body Mass Index Chart**

| Height (in.) | 49 | 51 | 53 | 55 | 57 | 59 | 61 | 63 | 65 | 67 | 69 | 71 | 73 | 75 | 77 | 79 | 81 | 83 |
|---|---|---|---|---|---|---|---|---|---|---|---|---|---|---|---|---|---|---|
| Weight (lb.) | | | | | | | | | | | | | | | | | | |
| 66 | 19 | 18 | 16 | 15 | 14 | 13 | 12 | 12 | 11 | 10 | 10 | 9 | 9 | 8 | 8 | 8 | 7 | 7 |
| 70 | 20 | 19 | 18 | 16 | 15 | 14 | 13 | 13 | 12 | 11 | 10 | 10 | 9 | 9 | 8 | 8 | 8 | 7 |
| 75 | 22 | 20 | 19 | 17 | 16 | 15 | 14 | 13 | 12 | 12 | 11 | 10 | 10 | 9 | 9 | 9 | 8 | 8 |
| 79 | 23 | 21 | 20 | 18 | 17 | 16 | 15 | 14 | 13 | 12 | 12 | 11 | 11 | 10 | 9 | 9 | 9 | 8 |
| 84 | 24 | 22 | 21 | 19 | 18 | 17 | 16 | 15 | 14 | 13 | 12 | 12 | 11 | 11 | 10 | 10 | 9 | 9 |
| 88 | 26 | 24 | 22 | 20 | 19 | 18 | 17 | 16 | 15 | 14 | 13 | 12 | 12 | 11 | 11 | 10 | 10 | 9 |
| 92 | 27 | 25 | 23 | 21 | 20 | 19 | 17 | 16 | 15 | 15 | 14 | 13 | 12 | 12 | 11 | 11 | 10 | 10 |
| 97 | 28 | 26 | 24 | 22 | 21 | 20 | 18 | 17 | 16 | 15 | 14 | 14 | 13 | 12 | 12 | 11 | 10 | 10 |
| 101 | 29 | 27 | 25 | 23 | 22 | 20 | 19 | 18 | 17 | 16 | 15 | 14 | 13 | 13 | 12 | 12 | 11 | 10 |
| 106 | 31 | 28 | 26 | 24 | 23 | 21 | 20 | 19 | 18 | 17 | 16 | 15 | 14 | 13 | 13 | 12 | 11 | 11 |
| 110 | 32 | 30 | 27 | 26 | 24 | 22 | 21 | 20 | 18 | 17 | 16 | 15 | 15 | 14 | 13 | 13 | 11 | 11 |
| 114 | 33 | 31 | 29 | 27 | 25 | 23 | 22 | 20 | 19 | 18 | 17 | 16 | 15 | 14 | 14 | 13 | 12 | 12 |
| 119 | 35 | 32 | 30 | 28 | 26 | 24 | 22 | 21 | 20 | 19 | 18 | 17 | 16 | 15 | 14 | 14 | 13 | 12 |
| 123 | 36 | 33 | 31 | 29 | 27 | 25 | 23 | 22 | 21 | 19 | 18 | 17 | 16 | 16 | 15 | 14 | 13 | 13 |
| 128 | 37 | 34 | 32 | 30 | 28 | 26 | 24 | 23 | 21 | 20 | 19 | 18 | 17 | 16 | 15 | 15 | 14 | 13 |
| 132 | 38 | 36 | 33 | 31 | 29 | 27 | 25 | 23 | 22 | 21 | 20 | 19 | 18 | 17 | 16 | 15 | 14 | 14 |
| 136 | 40 | 37 | 34 | 32 | 29 | 28 | 26 | 24 | 23 | 21 | 20 | 19 | 18 | 17 | 16 | 16 | 15 | 14 |
| 141 | 41 | 38 | 35 | 33 | 30 | 28 | 27 | 25 | 24 | 22 | 21 | 20 | 19 | 18 | 17 | 16 | 15 | 15 |
| 145 | 42 | 39 | 36 | 34 | 31 | 29 | 27 | 26 | 24 | 23 | 22 | 20 | 19 | 18 | 17 | 17 | 16 | 15 |
| 150 | 44 | 40 | 37 | 35 | 32 | 30 | 28 | 27 | 25 | 24 | 22 | 21 | 20 | 19 | 18 | 17 | 16 | 15 |
| 154 | 45 | 41 | 38 | 36 | 33 | 31 | 29 | 27 | 26 | 24 | 23 | 22 | 20 | 19 | 18 | 18 | 17 | 16 |
| 158 | 46 | 43 | 40 | 37 | 34 | 32 | 30 | 28 | 26 | 25 | 24 | 22 | 21 | 20 | 19 | 18 | 17 | 16 |
| 163 | 47 | 44 | 41 | 38 | 35 | 33 | 31 | 29 | 27 | 26 | 24 | 23 | 22 | 20 | 19 | 19 | 18 | 17 |
| 167 | 49 | 45 | 42 | 39 | 36 | 34 | 32 | 30 | 28 | 26 | 25 | 23 | 22 | 21 | 20 | 19 | 18 | 17 |
| 172 | 50 | 46 | 43 | 40 | 37 | 35 | 32 | 30 | 29 | 27 | 25 | 24 | 23 | 22 | 21 | 20 | 19 | 18 |
| 176 | 51 | 47 | 44 | 41 | 38 | 36 | 33 | 31 | 29 | 28 | 26 | 25 | 23 | 22 | 21 | 20 | 19 | 18 |
| 180 | 52 | 49 | 45 | 42 | 39 | 36 | 34 | 32 | 30 | 28 | 27 | 25 | 24 | 23 | 22 | 21 | 20 | 19 |
| 185 | 54 | 50 | 46 | 43 | 40 | 37 | 35 | 33 | 31 | 29 | 27 | 26 | 25 | 23 | 22 | 21 | 20 | 19 |
| 189 | 55 | 51 | 47 | 44 | 41 | 38 | 36 | 34 | 32 | 30 | 28 | 27 | 25 | 24 | 23 | 22 | 20 | 20 |
| 194 | 56 | 52 | 48 | 45 | 42 | 39 | 37 | 34 | 32 | 30 | 29 | 27 | 26 | 24 | 23 | 22 | 21 | 20 |
| 198 | 58 | 53 | 49 | 46 | 43 | 40 | 37 | 35 | 33 | 31 | 29 | 28 | 26 | 25 | 24 | 23 | 21 | 20 |
| 202 | 59 | 54 | 50 | 47 | 44 | 41 | 38 | 36 | 34 | 32 | 30 | 28 | 27 | 25 | 24 | 23 | 22 | 21 |
| 207 | 60 | 56 | 52 | 48 | 45 | 42 | 39 | 37 | 35 | 33 | 31 | 29 | 27 | 26 | 25 | 24 | 22 | 21 |
| 211 | 61 | 57 | 53 | 49 | 46 | 43 | 40 | 38 | 35 | 33 | 31 | 30 | 28 | 27 | 25 | 24 | 23 | 22 |
| 216 | 63 | 58 | 54 | 50 | 47 | 44 | 41 | 38 | 36 | 34 | 32 | 30 | 29 | 27 | 26 | 25 | 23 | 22 |
| 220 | 64 | 59 | 55 | 51 | 48 | 44 | 42 | 39 | 37 | 35 | 33 | 31 | 29 | 28 | 26 | 25 | 24 | 23 |
| 224 | 65 | 60 | 56 | 52 | 49 | 45 | 42 | 40 | 37 | 35 | 33 | 31 | 30 | 28 | 27 | 26 | 24 | 23 |
| 229 | 67 | 62 | 57 | 53 | 49 | 46 | 43 | 41 | 38 | 36 | 34 | 32 | 30 | 29 | 27 | 26 | 25 | 24 |
| 233 | 68 | 63 | 58 | 54 | 50 | 47 | 44 | 41 | 39 | 37 | 35 | 33 | 31 | 29 | 28 | 27 | 25 | 24 |
| 238 | 69 | 64 | 59 | 55 | 51 | 48 | 45 | 42 | 40 | 37 | 35 | 33 | 32 | 30 | 28 | 27 | 26 | 24 |
| 242 | 70 | 65 | 60 | 56 | 52 | 49 | 46 | 43 | 40 | 38 | 36 | 34 | 32 | 30 | 29 | 28 | 26 | 25 |
| 246 | 72 | 66 | 61 | 57 | 53 | 50 | 47 | 44 | 41 | 39 | 37 | 35 | 33 | 31 | 29 | 28 | 27 | 25 |
| 251 | 73 | 67 | 63 | 58 | 54 | 51 | 47 | 45 | 42 | 39 | 37 | 35 | 33 | 32 | 30 | 29 | 27 | 26 |
| 255 | 74 | 69 | 64 | 59 | 55 | 52 | 48 | 45 | 43 | 40 | 38 | 36 | 34 | 32 | 31 | 29 | 28 | 26 |
| 260 | 76 | 70 | 65 | 60 | 56 | 52 | 49 | 46 | 43 | 41 | 39 | 36 | 34 | 33 | 31 | 30 | 28 | 27 |
| 264 | 77 | 71 | 66 | 61 | 57 | 53 | 50 | 47 | 44 | 42 | 39 | 37 | 35 | 33 | 32 | 30 | 29 | 27 |
| 268 | 78 | 72 | 67 | 62 | 58 | 54 | 51 | 48 | 45 | 42 | 40 | 38 | 36 | 34 | 32 | 31 | 29 | 28 |
| 273 | 79 | 73 | 68 | 63 | 59 | 55 | 52 | 48 | 46 | 43 | 40 | 38 | 36 | 34 | 33 | 31 | 30 | 28 |
| 277 | 81 | 75 | 69 | 64 | 60 | 56 | 52 | 49 | 46 | 44 | 41 | 39 | 37 | 35 | 33 | 32 | 30 | 29 |
| 282 | 82 | 76 | 70 | 65 | 61 | 57 | 53 | 50 | 47 | 44 | 42 | 40 | 37 | 35 | 34 | 32 | 30 | 29 |
| 286 | 83 | 77 | 71 | 66 | 62 | 58 | 54 | 51 | 48 | 45 | 42 | 40 | 38 | 36 | 34 | 33 | 31 | 29 |
| 290 | 84 | 78 | 72 | 67 | 63 | 59 | 55 | 52 | 48 | 46 | 43 | 41 | 39 | 37 | 35 | 33 | 31 | 30 |
| 295 | 86 | 79 | 74 | 68 | 64 | 60 | 56 | 52 | 49 | 46 | 44 | 41 | 39 | 37 | 35 | 34 | 32 | 30 |
| 299 | 87 | 80 | 75 | 69 | 65 | 60 | 57 | 53 | 50 | 47 | 44 | 42 | 40 | 38 | 36 | 34 | 32 | 31 |
| 304 | 88 | 82 | 76 | 70 | 66 | 61 | 57 | 54 | 51 | 48 | 45 | 43 | 40 | 38 | 36 | 35 | 33 | 31 |
| 308 | 90 | 83 | 77 | 71 | 67 | 62 | 58 | 55 | 51 | 48 | 46 | 43 | 41 | 39 | 37 | 35 | 33 | 32 |
| 312 | 91 | 84 | 78 | 72 | 68 | 63 | 59 | 55 | 52 | 49 | 46 | 44 | 41 | 39 | 37 | 36 | 34 | 32 |

= Extremely obese.

= Obese;

= Increased health risks;

= Desirable;

= Underweight;

Note. Categories are based on value published by the Panel on Energy, Obesity, and Body Weight Standards, 1987, American Journal of Clinical

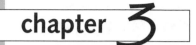

# Identifying Your Fitness Goals

### Edmund R. Burke, PhD

*O*ver the past 25 years, ever since the introduction of Dr. Kenneth Cooper's book, *Aerobics*, many individuals have focused on walking, running, cycling, swimming, and other types of aerobic activity as their only means of exercise. Unfortunately, this has led to many of these people neglecting other key components of fitness such as strength training, flexibility, and body composition. Many of us lack the strength to carry a full bag of groceries or the flexibility to pick up our shoes without bending at the knees. In addition, as we have aged, we have replaced muscle tissue with fat tissue.

Continuing work at the Cooper Institute for Aerobics Research is showing that in addition to the need to stress our cardiovascular system, more attention needs to be paid to building stronger muscles and increasing joint flexibility. This is necessary to achieve the benefits of balanced fitness: regular physical activity that includes strength training and flexibility (stretching) exercises in addition to aerobic conditioning. When developing your home fitness program, it is important that you develop all four components to achieve balanced fitness and thus optimal health and quality of life.

# COMPONENTS OF BALANCED FITNESS

Many people who are considering starting a balanced home fitness program still believe in the old no pain, no gain approach. They think they have to cycle or lift weights until they are overtired and their bodies ache. What those who hold to this outdated idea of fitness don't realize is that, using proper guidelines, in a short time any initial tiredness or soreness will be replaced by increased energy for work and recreation and an increased sense of well-being.

Since 1978, the American College of Sports Medicine (ACSM) has influenced the medical and scientific communities with its position statement on "The Recommended Quantity and Quality of Exercise for Developing and Maintaining Fitness in Healthy Adults." For the first time since 1978, the ACSM has revised its recommendations on exercise for healthy adults. A new paper published in 1991 expands and revises advice on cardiovascular fitness and body composition and now recommends that you add resistance training. This is new information for those of us whose attempts to maintain fitness have been limited to cycling, running, swimming, watching our body weight, and controlling our diet.

Balanced fitness can do more to ensure a long, healthy life than just about anything else known to the medical community today. It's never too late to start a fitness program, but ideally, you should build strong muscles, flexibility, and a strong cardiovascular system early in life and enter the later years with your physical potential at its maximum.

## CARDIOVASCULAR FITNESS

The new ACSM guidelines repeat the recommendations on duration, intensity, frequency, and various modes of aerobic activity but with slight changes. The recommended duration is now 20 to 60 minutes versus the previous minimum of 15 minutes.

Intensity of exercise can be determined using two methods. The first and most familiar is use of target heart rate. The guidelines state that you should aim to work at 60 to 90 percent of your maximum heart rate (MHR = 220 − your age), or 50 to 85 percent of your maximal oxygen capacity (determined by doing a stress test on a stationary bicycle or treadmill at a medical facility). See "Determining Your Target Heart Rate Zone," p. 40.

Duration is dependent upon the intensity of the activity; those who like to work at a lower intensity should work out longer. Low- to moderate-intensity cycling, stepping, walking, or cross-country skiing is best for most adults because higher intensity workouts can lead to increased risk of injury and it is easier to adhere to this type of exercise routine. Beginners can achieve a significant training effect from low-intensity workouts. If you're already fit and want to improve, gradually increase your intensity.

Again, the type of activity should include any exercise that uses large muscle groups and is rhythmical and aerobic in nature, such as stationary cycling, treadmill walking or running, stair climbing, or indoor skiing. Other activities could include swimming, indoor cycling, or walking. These activities need to be done 3 to 5 days per week.

After several weeks of aerobic conditioning, certain changes become apparent. What was once a barely attainable level of exercise now becomes quite easy. Whereas cycling or running at a certain pace or speed previously may have caused your heart rate to go up to 135 beats per minute, that pace can now be achieved at a lower heart rate. In short, your heart is becoming stronger, larger, and more efficient, and your body is able to do the same work with less strain.

Regardless of your maximum average heart rate or your target heart rate, you should consult with your physician or with a sports medicine expert to establish, with precision, the rates that are right for you, your age, and your medical and physical condition. This is especially important if you are over 35, have been sedentary for several years, are overweight, or have a history of heart disease in your family.

## MUSCULAR STRENGTH

The new guidelines have added resistance training because the ACSM now recognizes the increasing importance of maintaining strength as a health benefit as we get older. The rationale for adding strength training to the guidelines is the result of a 10-year follow-up study of master runners (along with other studies). Those who continued to train aerobically without upper body exercise maintained their body's oxygen-transporting capacity over the years but lost about 4.5 pounds of lean body mass; those who included strength training in their program maintained their lean body mass along with their aerobic capacity after 10 years of aging.

If you scored below average on the push-up test or low on the bench press test, you should consider purchasing free weights or a multi-station weight machine as part of your home fitness gym.

The guidelines also show that consistent resistance training helps maintain bone and muscle mass as we get older. For women, strength training (along with the aerobic work) may also protect against postmenopausal bone loss and osteoporosis in later years.

The guidelines recommend that two strength training sessions per week be added to your workout schedule. The new ACSM guidelines recommend one set of 8 to 12 repetitions of 8 to 10 strength

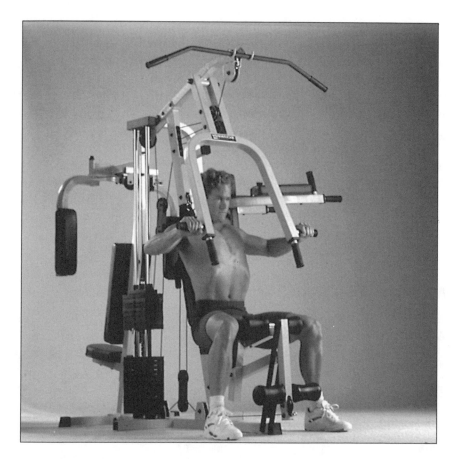

exercises of your major muscle groups per session as the minimum requirement. A complete detailed strength training program will be outlined later in this book. If weights or other resistance training devices are not available, add calisthenics to your program.

## FLEXIBILITY

To be in total balance, it is important to have flexibility. By incorporating basic stretches into your fitness routine, you can prevent and alleviate most muscle soreness and strains.

The best reason to stretch is simply that it feels good—if done correctly. The key is to relax and listen to your body. If you had difficulty scoring in the average range on the sit-and-reach test, you will need to work on loosening up your muscles, tendons, and ligaments. You may also consider adding additional flexibility sessions to your fitness program each week. A good time to add these sessions is during the evening while watching television or playing with the kids.

Proper stretching reduces muscle tension and allows for freer movement. Extreme flexibility is not the goal and can often lead to overstretching and injury. As Bob Anderson, the author of *Stretching*, will show in chapter 4, the key is to not push yourself. Let your body tell you your limits.

Although not part of the ACSM guidelines, flexibility is important for you to perform tasks that require reaching or twisting and turning your body. Hip flexibility, for example, is important to preventing lower back pain. The stretching exercises included in chapter 4 will help improve the flexibility of your body's major joints.

## BODY COMPOSITION

Body composition is an important component of health-related fitness. Good body composition results from aerobic activity, strength training, and proper diet. Your everyday caloric balance will determine whether you will gain or lose weight from day to day. Caloric balance refers to the difference between the calories you take in from food and your caloric expenditure, or the amount of energy you put out in daily activities, work, or exercise.

If you scored in the "Increased Health Risks" zone or lower on the body composition test, it is important to begin a weight loss program that incorporates diet and exercise. Body weight is lost when caloric expenditure exceeds caloric intake from food or when caloric intake is less than caloric expenditure during work or exercise. It is a known physiological fact that 1 pound of fat is equal to 3,500 calories of energy. Although shifts in caloric balance will be accompanied by changes in body weight, how your body loses weight varies depending on the type of weight loss program you undertake. For example, low-calorie diets cause a substantial loss of water and lean body tissue such as muscle. In contrast, an exercise-induced negative caloric balance results in a weight loss of primarily fat stores.

If you were to add a resistance training component to your program, you might also see a slight increase in weight due to a gain in muscle mass, whereas an aerobic-based program usually results in a maintenance of muscle mass. Although both approaches to weight loss are effective, aerobic activity is usually found to be more effective because metabolism is sustained for longer periods of time and energy. Expenditure is greater with activities that use large muscle groups, such as walking, cycling, cross-county skiing, and so on.

Follow these guidelines when engaging in a weight loss program that combines exercise and caloric restriction:

- Ensure that you are consuming at least 1,000 to 1,200 calories per day in a balanced diet. You need to consume calories for healthy everyday bodily functions.

- You should not exceed a 500- to 1,000-calorie-per-day negative caloric balance, combining both caloric restriction and exercise. This will result in a gradual weight loss without loss of lean body weight (muscle). You should not lose more than 2 pounds per week on a diet.

- Include an exercise program that will expend at least 300 calories or more per day. This is best accomplished with exercise of low intensity and long duration. Many pieces of home fitness equipment give estimates of calories burned while exercising. Remember these are approximate calories burned; exact amounts will depend on body size, type of exercise, intensity, and duration.

- Add resistance training to your program to add muscle mass. Muscle cells are more active than fat cells and will help you burn more calories per day.

- Include use of behavior modification techniques to identify and eliminate bad diet and eating habits.

You should strive to burn between 300 and 500 calories per exercise session and 1,000 to 2,000 calories per week in exercise. Remember that sustained aerobic activities that use large muscle groups will cause the greatest energy expenditure.

---

### Resistance Training and Weight Loss

A recent study at the University of Massachusetts Medical Center compared weight loss and body changes in 65 subjects. Some subjects just dieted, some dieted and did aerobic exercise, some dieted and took part in strength training, and some dieted and took part in both strength and aerobic training.
The results:

- The diet-only group lost 9 pounds, between 11 and 25 percent of which was lean body mass (muscle).

- Those who dieted and did aerobic exercise lost 10 pounds, 99 percent of which was fat.

- Most successful were the diet and strength training group and the group that took part in all three activities. The first group lost 9 pounds, 109 percent from fat, and the three-method group lost 13 pounds, 104 percent from fat. How can you lose more than 100 percent fat? By gaining lean body mass.

---

If overweight or obese, you may want to keep the intensity even lower than 60 percent of MHR to keep the risk of orthopedic injuries at a minimum. Non–weight-bearing activities such as stationary cycling may be considered for this group, or for those who suffer from orthopedic or arthritis problems.

Wayne Westcott, a contributor to this book, recently conducted a study on exercise and weight control at the YMCA where he serves as fitness director. Seventy-two overweight men and women were placed into two groups. Both groups followed a recommended diet of 60 percent carbohydrate, 20 percent fat, and 20 percent protein. Both groups exercised 30 minutes per day, 3 days per week, for 8 weeks, but 22 subjects followed a program of 30 minutes of aerobic activity and the other 50 performed 15 minutes of aerobic

| Table 3.1 | Exercise Group Results | | | |
| --- | --- | --- | --- | --- |
| Subjects | Number | Body weight changes | Fat weight changes | Muscle weight changes |
| Endurance exercise only | 22 | − 3.5 lb | − 3.0 lb | − 0.5 lb |
| Endurance and strength exercise | 50 | − 8.0 lb | − 10.0 lb | + 2.0 lb |

exercise and 15 minutes of resistance training. The results are shown in Table 3.1.

The group that combined both aerobic exercise and strength training showed the greatest changes in body composition. Most subjects lost fat and gained in muscle mass.

# EXERCISE GUIDELINES

Duration, intensity, and frequency of training stimulate the aerobic training effect. Any training performed below the ACSM guidelines will not be sufficient to produce the aerobic training effect. Conversely, exercising at more than the recommended levels will not significantly increase the aerobic training effect (although athletes training for competition need to exercise more to be competitive). It is important to remember not to overdo it; your body needs adequate recovery from a hard workout.

In general, endurance training for fewer than 2 days per week, at less than 60 percent of MHR, for fewer than 20 minutes per day, and without a well-rounded resistance and flexibility program is inadequate for developing and maintaining fitness in healthy adults. It is just that simple.

Now you may have read that the National Centers for Disease Control and the ACSM recommend just getting up and moving for

30 minutes a day. Whether by walking, gardening, cleaning the house, or taking the stairs instead of the elevator, it's the movement that counts. However, they based this fitness theory on the goal of achieving the "health" benefits of exercise, and established it knowing that only about 20% of the population exercises on a regular basis. The get-up-and-get-moving principle may be a good starting point for many individuals, but we want to take you beyond the basics, improve your cardiorespiratory fitness, and add muscular strength and flexibility to your fitness program.

Keep in mind that the ACSM recommendations are guidelines for the average person, not for a champion athlete training for the Olympics. An appropriate warm-up and cool-down, which should include flexibility exercises, is also recommended. Although many of you will need to train with more mileage and at a greater intensity to race competitively, the important factor to remember for most people is that if they follow the ACSM guidelines of physical activity, they will attain increased physical and health benefits at the lowest risk. Table 3.2 outlines the guidelines.

If followed, the ACSM guidelines can result in permanent lifestyle changes for most individuals. The good news is that, with the right approach, exercising at home can and should be pleasant. You can combine strength training, aerobic exercise, and flexibility activities that you enjoy to gain valuable health benefits.

**Table 3.2   Exercise Fitness Guidelines**

|  | Strength training | Aerobic exercise | Stretching |
|---|---|---|---|
| Frequency | 2 to 3 sessions/week | 3 to 5 sessions/week | 3 to 6 sessions/week |
| Intensity | 8-12 repetitions until fatigued | 60-90 percent of MHR | "Easy" feeling stretch |
| Time | 20-40 min | 20-60 min | 10 min |
| Type | 8-10 exercises | Any rhythmical activity | 10 stretches |

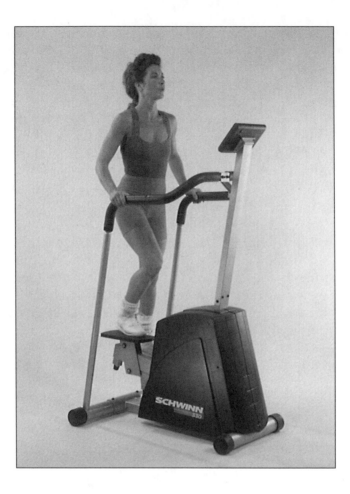

# DETERMINING YOUR TARGET HEART RATE ZONE

For maximum training benefit, you need to exercise within a precise target heart rate range. Although competitive athletes train at 80 to 100 percent of MHR, most noncompetitive athletes get very good aerobic training effects by working out at 70 to 80 percent of maximum. If you are interested primarily in weight loss, you should exercise five or six times per week at 60 to 70 percent of maximum. If your goal is to reduce your risk of chronic disease such as heart disease, exercising at 50 to 60 percent of maximum a few times a week should be adequate.

All types of exercise are equally effective when your heart rate is maintained within your target zone. By checking your heart rate from time to time, you can adjust the intensity of your exercise as needed. A bonus of heart rate monitoring is that it allows you to derive the same cardiovascular fitness benefit from all the equipment in your home gym. Once you know what level of intensity produces your target heart rate for each type of equipment or routine, you can adjust the intensity of your workout to equalize the effect.

To develop your target heart rate zone, you must first determine your maximum heart rate. The best time to do that is while performing at maximum effort on a stationary bike, stair climber, treadmill, or indoor cross-country ski machine. Simply record your heart rate several times while working at maximum effort, such as when going all out on a stationary bicycle or during a hard session of stair climbing. Caution: Only attempt this if you are healthy and have not experienced undue discomfort or lightheadedness while exercising.

If such a stressful test is not reasonable, you can estimate your maximum heart rate using the following formula, which has been well-established for reliability: Subtract your age from the number 220. Your target heart rate zone for aerobic conditioning will be 70 to 80 percent of the resulting number (see Table 3.3). For example, the estimated maximum heart rate for a 45-year-old would be 175 (220 − 45 = 175), and the target heart rate zone for aerobic training would be 123 to 140 beats per minute (70 to 80 percent of 175).

Table 3.3  Predicted Target Heart Rate Zones for Different Ages

| Age | Maximum predicted heart rate | Aerobic target zone: 70-80% |
|-----|------------------------------|------------------------------|
| 20 | 200 | 140-160 |
| 25 | 195 | 137-156 |
| 30 | 190 | 133-152 |
| 35 | 185 | 130-148 |
| 40 | 180 | 126-144 |
| 45 | 175 | 123-140 |
| 50 | 170 | 119-136 |
| 55 | 165 | 116-132 |
| 60 | 160 | 112-128 |

There are three primary heart rate training zones. The first is often referred to as the "fat-burning zone" because the intensity is sufficient to require your body to use fat as the primary fuel source for the exercise. You should exercise at 60 to 70 percent of your maximum heart rate to achieve this level of intensity. While working out in this and the other zones, your heart rate should fall somewhere between these two figures. If you are just beginning an exercise program or want to lose weight, you should concentrate on maintaining your heart rate in this zone for 20 to 30 minutes per day, 3 to 5 days per week. If you scored below average in the Rockport Walking Test, you should consider exercising in this zone for several weeks

In the second zone, known as the "aerobic exercise zone" or "target heart rate zone," you should exercise at 70 to 80 percent of MHR. Training in this zone helps build aerobic endurance and constructs a base upon which you can progressively add more demanding workouts as your cardiovascular fitness increases. Exercise at this intensity only if you scored average to above average in the Rockport Walking Test.

Training in the third zone, referred to as anaerobic training, can help increase both your speed and your tolerance for the buildup of lactic acid, the primary waste product of anaerobic metabolism in your muscles. This type of workout, which ranges from 80 to 100 percent of MHR, usually consists of short, hard sprints or repeated incline running on a treadmill.

Varied training in all three zones will increase fitness, improve performance, and add energy to your life. Most training programs use a combination of intensities to increase performance capacity, according to J.T. Kearney, PhD, Senior Exercise Physiologist at the U.S. Olympic Training Center. Kearney suggests that it is important to monitor intensity. There are many different ways to do this, but monitoring heart rate response is the simplest, most convenient, and least expensive method.

Using your fingers to take your pulse is not as convenient or reliable as using some of the extremely accurate heart rate monitors available today. Heart rate monitors with a wireless receiver and chest band do not interfere with your ability to exercise on any piece of home equipment and are as accurate as an EKG machine. The heart rate is transmitted to the wrist receiver for viewing. Some heart rate monitors even allow you to program your target heart rate zone and audibly alert you when you rise above or fall below that zone. Some electronic bikes, steppers, and ski machines are equipped with compatible receivers and interactive software that automatically adjust the intensity to keep your heart rate at an effective level. Heart rate monitors will be discussed further in chapter 14.

Type of exercise also affects your heart rate. Those that use more and larger muscles raise the heart rate more than those that use fewer and smaller muscles. Running on a treadmill raises your heart rate more than cycling, so you will adjust your workload differently for a stationary bicycle than for a treadmill to achieve a target heart rate.

# BALANCED WORKOUTS

To achieve balance, all of your home workouts should include three phases: (a) Warm-up, (b) an aerobic and/or strength routine, and cool-down.

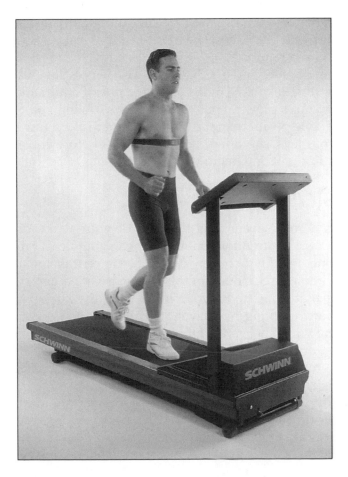

Together, exercise and recovery constitute fitness conditioning; omit either and you invite injury and minimize benefits. Our bodies and minds become stronger and more efficient in response to use and exercise. Overuse and overload will cause breakdown. The secret is to know when you are pushing too much or too little. Monitoring your heart rate tells you how much to exercise and when to rest.

## WARM-UP

A good warm-up will help you perform better and will decrease the aches and pains most people experience. The warm-up prepares your muscles for exercise and allows your oxygen supply to ready itself for what's to come. Studies show that muscles perform best when they are warmer than normal body temperature. Exercises that can be used for warm-up include cycling, walking, or skiing slowly until you begin to break a light sweat. This usually takes about 5 to 10 minutes, or if using target heart rate, until it reaches about 50 to 60 percent of maximum.

Stretching before and after exercise also serves several purposes. By promoting flexibility, it decreases the risk of injury and soreness. It also enhances physical performance by allowing you to maintain a comfortable position on the bicycle longer. Take a few minutes to stretch your legs, shoulders, and lower back before you get on your home equipment and begin your warm-up.

## AEROBIC/STRENGTH EXERCISE

Vigorous aerobic exercise is the core of your workout program. Exercise must be strenuous enough to raise your heart rate into your target zone, usually between 70 and 80 percent of maximum. Cycling, or any exercise done in this range, is called aerobic exercise, meaning that your body, your heart, and the various exercising muscles are working at a level at which oxygen can be utilized. Exercising with a heart rate monitor provides constant visible feedback (and on some models, audible feedback) as to your heart rate while exercising and allows you to stay within your selected target heart rate zone.

In addition to aerobic exercise, the ACSM recommends that healthy adults perform a minimum of 8 to 10 strength exercises involving the major muscle groups two times per week. At least one set of 8 to 12 repetitions to near fatigue should be completed during each session.

These recommendations are based on two factors:

- Most people aren't likely to adhere to an aerobic workout session that lasts more than 60 minutes. The regimen outlined above can be completed in 30 minutes or less, and when combined with 30 minutes of aerobic activity and flexibility, gives you a balanced workout.

- Although more frequent and intense training is likely to build greater strength, the difference is usually very small.

## COOL-DOWN

The cool-down enables your body's cardiovascular system to gradually return to normal, preferably over a 5- to 10-minute period. Bringing your workout to an abrupt halt can cause lightheadedness because blood will pool in your legs if you stop working abruptly. Lower your exercise intensity gradually over a period of a few minutes. When your heart rate has returned to below 60 percent of maximum, you can stop exercising.

Always keep in mind that warm-up and cool-down are as important as the activity phase. Both can prevent common injuries.

# A NEW AGE OF FITNESS

The combination of aerobic exercise, strength training, flexibility, and weight control is referred to as balanced fitness. It has broad implications for us as individuals and as a society. It will make you healthier and increase your self-esteem and self-confidence. It will reduce your medical costs and increase your work productivity.

Periodically retake the tests in chapter 2 to chart your gains in fitness—what better form of motivation is there than to see the progress you are making?

Now that you've seen the multidimensional scope of fitness, in the next chapters you will examine how to stretch properly, how to use your equipment correctly and safely, and how to develop home fitness programs—and enjoy your first step in making home exercise a part of your life.

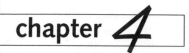

# Stretching

**Bob Anderson, BS**

*F*lexibility, the ability of your joints to move through their full range of motion, is one of the key components in your balanced fitness program, along with cardiovascular endurance and muscular strength. The way to improve or maintain your flexibility is to stretch.

Stretching is not just for athletes. More than anyone, active people need the relief from muscle tension and stiffness that stretching will provide. Numerous studies have shown that as we get older, our muscles lose elasticity, and stretching helps maintain our flexibility and may enhance our physical performance. When done properly and on a regular basis, stretching feels good.

## HEALTH AND FLEXIBILITY

One of the most obvious signs associated with aging is reduced flexibility. For many older individuals, range of motion becomes so restricted that they may be afraid of becoming injured when entering an exercise program. Luckily, inflexibility can be reversed in the elderly. One study compared the joint stiffness of a group of 20 young men (15 to 19 years of age) and 20 elderly men (63 to 88 years of age) and found that both groups could reverse joint stiffness with equal ease. Several other studies have shown that almost anyone, regardless of age, can improve flexibility by stretching.

Lack of flexibility can create poor posture, resulting in increased mechanical imbalances in the hips, neck, shoulders, and back. These imbalances pull body segments out of line, causing stress, strain, and, even worse, chronic changes in posture. The resulting muscular tension can put tremendous strain on ligaments and tendons. Inflexibility in the shoulders and upper back can lead to a humpbacked spine (kyphosis) and possibly reduced respiratory capacity. Tight muscles in the hips, the back of the legs, and the lower back can rotate the hips forward, resulting in excessive curvature of the lower back (lordosis), chronic lower back pain, and pain in the buttocks and thighs (sciatica).

Additionally, tight calf muscles can place undue stress on the foot, leading to a variety of orthopedic problems, including painful Achilles tendinitis. Remember, being flexible is not just for athletes. It can help provide relief from everyday muscle tension and stiffness, prevent muscular injury, and is also crucial for proper posture.

Stretching also affects your mind as well as your body. When completed slowly and with focus, stretching can be an excellent stress-reduction tool. This may be why so many individuals sign up for yoga classes.

Several studies have shown that a stretching and breathing routine can be as effective as other means of relaxation but at the same time can increase one's perception of physical and mental alertness and energy. In addition, it has been reported that stretching can help tense individuals reduce muscle tension and anxiety, as well as lower their breathing rate and blood pressure.

# STRETCHING DURING YOUR WORKOUT

Stretching and warm-up are two different things. You should stretch gently before you warm up prior to your exercise session. It prepares your muscles for exercise. If you wish, you may want to complete a light warm-up before your stretch, such as a minute or two on the bike, treadmill, or stepper.

After stretching, you can begin your formal warm-up. Start by walking on the treadmill, riding a stationary bicycle, or doing a short session on the stair climber at a low intensity. Warming up prepares you for exercise by gradually increasing your heart rate and blood flow and by raising the temperature of your muscles, ligaments, and tendons, all of which are vital for optimal functioning and increased elasticity of your muscles and connective tissue.

But the trick is to stretch properly. Studies show that you should stretch 3 to 6 days a week to increase your flexibility. For maintaining flexibility, 3 days is probably adequate.

Cool down at the end of your workout by doing a scaled-down version of your main exercise session. Get your heart rate down toward your resting rate. Stretch for a few minutes afterward to help reduce muscle soreness and stiffness. Complete several of the same stretches you used before exercising.

## ✔ TIPS FOR STRETCHING

Try to stretch several times per week to help maintain your flexibility. If you are injured or have a disability, your physician or trained medical personnel should be consulted.

Optimally, you should stretch slowly. Do not bounce, and do not push the stretch to the point of pain. Pain is a sign that you are stretching improperly. Most injuries occur when you push too hard or too fast. Keep your hands, feet, shoulders, and jaw relaxed as you stretch. Tension will hamper your stretching.

Move slowly into the stretch. Stretch to the point where you feel mild tension, then relax and hold the stretch for 5 to 15 seconds for most stretches. This easy stretch reduces muscular tightness and readies the muscles for the developmental stretch.

Move slowly into the developmental phase, stretching a fraction further until you feel minor tension, and hold for an additional 15 seconds. Remember, no bouncing.

When possible, stretch before your exercise session. You may also wish to stretch between exercises or when switching from one piece of equipment to another.

Breathe slowly and naturally. Do not hold your breath while stretching.

# 10 BALANCED STRETCHES

What follows are suggested stretches that can be added to your home fitness program. It will take about 5 minutes to complete the routine after you've learned the stretches. I have included more stretches than you may be able to complete during each session, and if you spend more than 30 seconds on any stretch, you may have to cut out a few to keep your stretching to 5 minutes. If you have time, stretch for a few minutes longer or repeat several of the stretches. Your body will appreciate it.

I believe that the more stretches you learn, the more you'll enjoy stretching. Eventually, you'll wonder how you lived without it.

## SITTING GROIN STRETCH

**Starting Position:** Sit on the floor with the soles of your feet together; hold onto your toes and feet.

**Movement:** Gently pull forward, bending from the hips; hold for 10 to 30 seconds; do not bounce, and breathe slowly and deeply.

**Muscles Emphasized:** Lower back and groin.

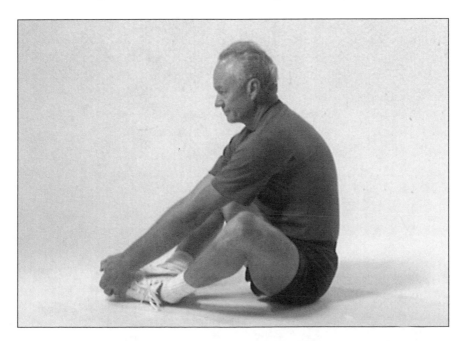

# WALL STRETCH

**Starting Position:** Stand slightly away from a wall or other stable object and lean on it with forearms, your head resting on your hands; place your right foot in front of you, leg bent, and your left leg straight behind you.

**Movement:** Slowly move your hips forward until you feel an easy stretch in the calf of your left leg; keep your heel flat and your toes pointed straight ahead; hold for 10 to 20 seconds; do not bounce, and do not hold your breath. Repeat on the other side.

**Muscles Emphasized:** Calf and Achilles tendon.

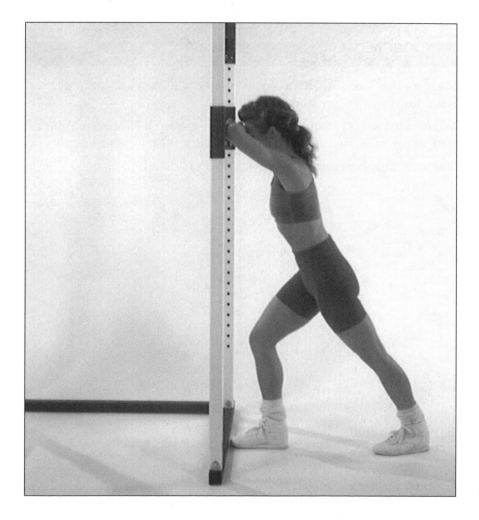

# OPPOSITE-HAND, OPPOSITE-FOOT QUAD STRETCH

**Starting Position:** Stand slightly away from a wall or other stable object and place your right hand on the wall for support.

**Movement:** Standing straight, grasp the top of your right foot with your left hand, pull your heel toward your buttocks, and hold for 10 to 20 seconds. Repeat on the other side.

**Muscles Emphasized:** Thigh.

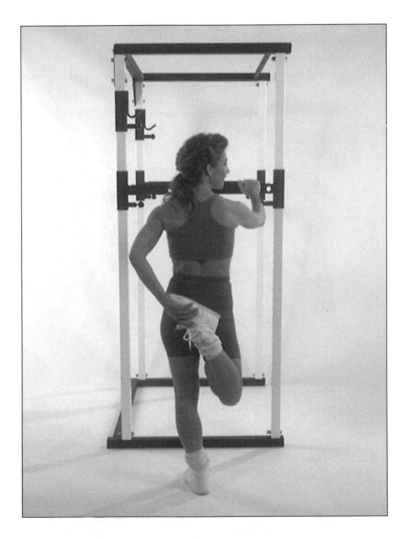

## SPRINTER'S STRETCH

**Starting Position:** From a kneeling position, move one leg forward until the knee is directly over the ankle and place the knee of the other leg behind, resting on the floor. Avoid the common mistake of hyperextending the knee past the ankle, as shown in the photo below.

**Movement:** Lower the front of the hip directly downward until you feel an easy stretch; hold for 10 to 20 seconds. Repeat on the other side.

**Muscles Emphasized:** Front of hip (iliopsoas) and lower back (excellent for the lower back).

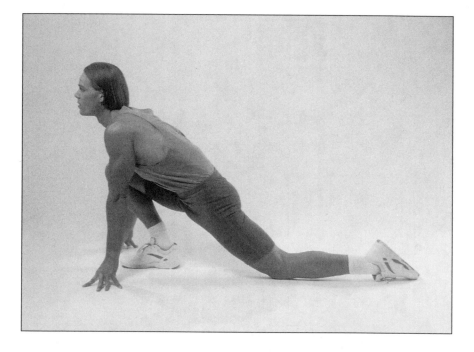

# LYING HAMSTRING

**Starting Position:** Lie on the floor and bend your left knee, keeping your foot flat; keep your lower back flat on the floor.

**Movement:** Lift right leg straight up from the hip and then lower it; hold for 10 to 20 seconds and repeat on the other side.

**Muscles Emphasized:** Hamstrings and calf.

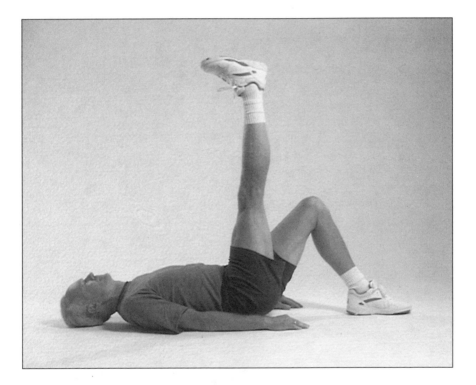

## UPWARD REACH

**Starting Position:** Interlace your fingers above your head, palms facing upward.

**Movement:** Push your arms slightly back and up and breathe easily; hold for 10 to 20 seconds.

**Muscles Emphasized:** Arms, back, and shoulders (excellent for slumping shoulders).

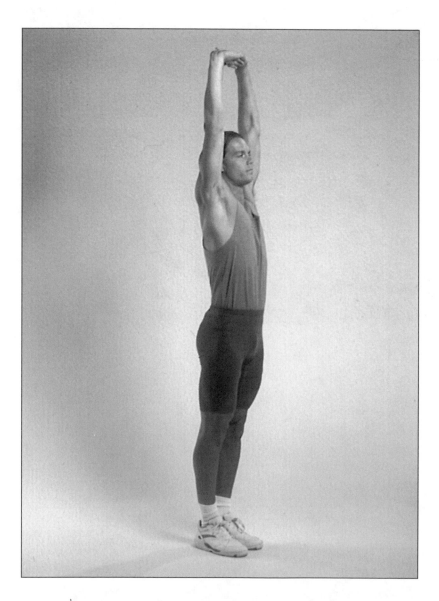

# UPPER ARM PULLOVER

**Starting Position:** Keep your knees slightly flexed while standing or sitting with your arms overhead, and hold your elbow with the hand of the opposite arm.

**Movement:** Gently pull your elbow behind your head as you slowly lean to the side until a mild stretch is felt and hold for 10 to 15 seconds. Repeat on the other side.

**Muscles Emphasized:** Back of arms, top of shoulders, and waist.

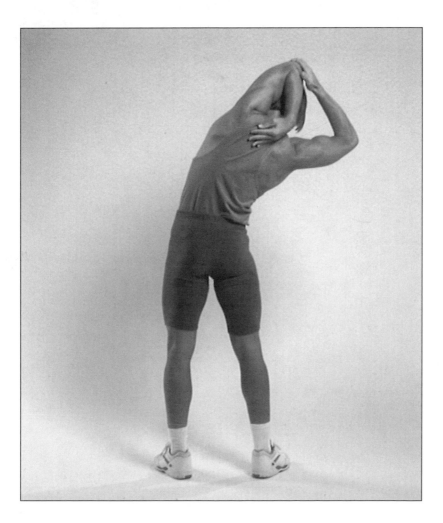

## STANDING ROTATION

**Starting Position:** Stand with your hands on your hips; keep your knees slightly bent.

**Movement:** Gently twist your torso at the waist until a stretch is felt and hold for 10 to 15 seconds. Repeat on the other side.

**Muscles Emphasized:** Middle of back.

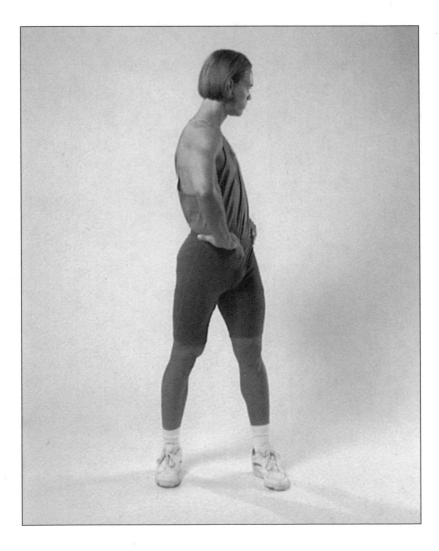

## ELONGATION

**Starting Position:** Lie on the floor; extend your arms overhead, keeping your legs straight.

**Movement:** Reach your arms and legs in opposite directions. Stretch for 5 seconds and relax.

**Muscles Emphasized:** Shoulders, arms, hands, feet, and ankles.

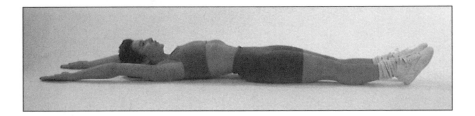

## WILLIAM'S STRETCH

**Starting Position:** Lie on the floor with your legs straight or with one leg bent (option).

**Movement:** Gently pull your left knee to your chest and hold for 10 to 30 seconds, then relax. Repeat with the other leg.

**Muscles Emphasized:** Lower back, hips, and hamstrings.

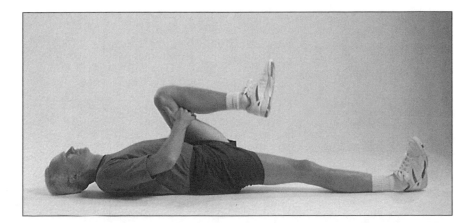

# STAYING LOOSE

Flexibility training should be a fundamental part of any balanced exercise program. Emphasis should be placed on proper body position, form, and execution of each stretch. When done correctly and regularly, stretching can be very enjoyable and relaxing. With so much attention now being paid to designing programs that enhance the interaction of mind, body, and spirit, flexibility training is an integral part of your fitness program.

# chapter 5

# Using Multistation Weight Machines

### Edmund R. Burke, PhD

*B*uying a multistation home gym is no longer simply a matter of deciding where the machine will go in your home. You are now faced with choosing the type of resistance (isotonic or isokinetic) and the form of resistance (traditional iron weight stacks, pneumatic, elastic bands, hydraulic cylinders). The good news is that in the moderate price category—between $1,000 and $2,500, or roughly membership dues for 2 years at the majority of quality health clubs—there has never been such a variety of well-engineered machines available to the home market.

Why choose a multistation gym? To put it simply, availability and space. Most of today's multipurpose gyms give you an impressive amount of equipment per square foot compared to free weights. A well-designed home gym will require approximately 50 to 70 square feet of floor space. Achieving the same workout using free weights and the necessary benches and racks could require up to 100 square feet or more.

Availability is the deciding factor for many exercisers. Multistation gyms allow you to complete a workout in very little time because placing plates on a barbell or dumbbell and moving benches and racks are eliminated from your program. Another major consideration for those working out at home is safety. Most multistation gyms eliminate the need for spotters—not to mention the possibility of dropping weights on the floor. The biggest advances in home gyms in the last few years have come in design improvement.

There are four fundamental types of home gym equipment: weight stack, hydraulic, pneumatic, and rods.

## WEIGHT STACK MACHINES

Essentially, these are mechanized free weights that allow you to lift specific amounts of weight plates by pulling or pushing on a bar or

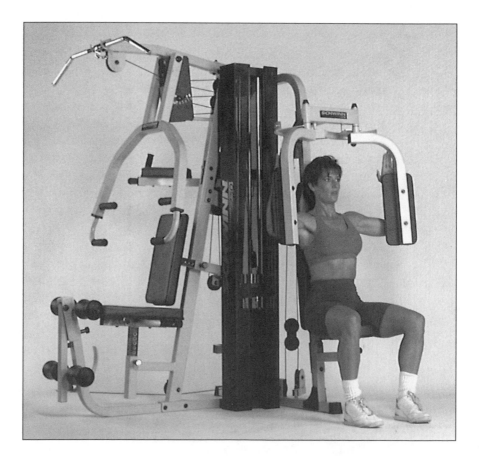

handle attached to a system of pulleys or a lever system. Pulleys should be 4 to 4-1/2 inches in diameter and made of good-quality plastic or fiberglass-reinforced nylon. Smaller pulleys put more stress on the cables and shorten their life. The cables themselves should be 2,000-pound tensile strength with quality nylon or rubber coating. Check the weight plates for quality of finish and consistency of shape—poor quality could indicate that the plates are not accurately weighted. Pivot points for levers should use quality bushings or ball bearings.

Check out the machine for danger zones such as open weight stacks. Many companies now shield or cover their weight stacks to keep fingers from getting pinched and to keep large amounts of weight from harming anyone. If you want the feel of metal against metal, the Schwinn® Home Trainer 730 with three workstations provides just about every possible workout option one would need at home.

Weightstrap machines, which are similar to weight stack machines, will be familiar to all TV viewers who watch ESPN and CNN and see Soloflex advertisements (around $1,000). Resistance is supplied by

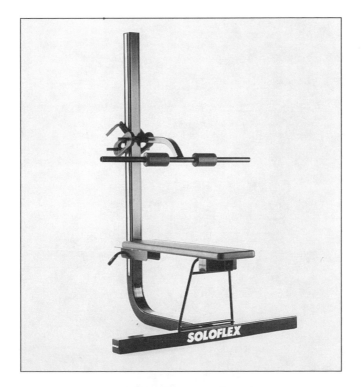

weightstraps attached between the machine's lever arm and frame. To increase resistance, you add more weightstraps, iron plates, or some combination of the two.

These types of machines offer traditional isotonic weight resistance—the positive/negative strength training method associated with free weights. In addition, Soloflex's patented floating barbell arm prevents the user's stronger side from "cheating" and helping the weaker side to lift the weight—one of the main advantages of free weight equipment.

# HYDRAULIC EQUIPMENT

Hydraulic machines use fluid to provide two-way positive resistance for strengthening and toning. The accommodating style of resistance matches the user's force curve through the range of motion. In other words, the same 15 pounds on another machine may

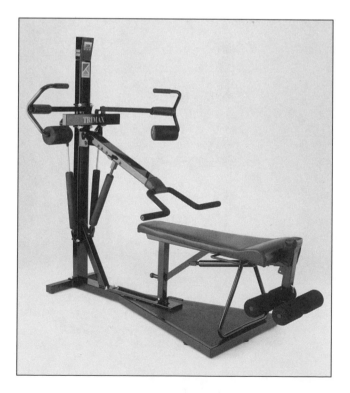

vary in weight during lifting, but with a hydraulic machine, the user's capabilities are matched throughout the exercise.

Beginning at zero resistance, hydraulic machines promise a full workout on stations such as a leg extender or triceps curl. For example, in a bench press, you can constantly pull and push instead of allowing for negative resistance while lowering the bar.

A new machine, the Trimax (around $1,400), employs pneumatic or accommodating resistance so that the harder you explode into the exercise, the greater the workload. The resistance works in both directions.

# PNEUMATIC EQUIPMENT

Using air within cylinders to create resistance, the pneumatic machine is ideal for strength training, toning, weight loss, and for a low-impact workout that's easy on the joints. As with a shock absorber on your car, you can change the resistance on a cylinder by turning an

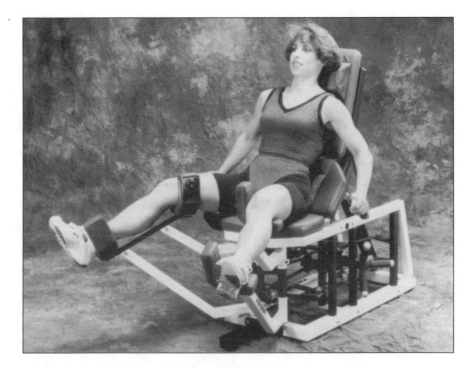

adjustment knob on one end or by pushing a button or footpad. Thus, you don't need to stop your workout to change pins or weight plates. Kaiser Physical Fitness is one of the largest manufacturers of pneumatic equipment for both the health club and home gym.

# RODS

Bow-Flex, Inc., of Vancouver, Washington, makes three models of multigyms ranging in price from $600 to $900 that use flexible rods to provide resistance. To increase resistance, the user simply hooks more of the rods, which come in varying weights, onto a cable.

# PURCHASING CONSIDERATIONS

The background research on multistation equipment should begin in your own home—make sure the ceiling is high enough to accommodate the particular unit you're thinking about purchasing. In addition, if you are really tight for space, consider a machine that offers a vertical bench press and a standing instead of prone leg curl. And remember, you get what you pay for in home gyms. Generally, moderately priced multistation machines don't have quality components, are not biomechanically designed, are not stable, and just don't have the feel of higher priced units. Conversely, do not overbuy. A higher priced machine may be too much equipment for your needs—and the additional money would be better spent on a treadmill or stationary bike.

The key is to find a home gym that fits you and the other members of your family for all exercises with a minimum of adjustment. Remember, convenience is a primary reason for owning a multistation gym. Machine positions should not be difficult to change.

Whatever type of machine you choose, be sure to check its overall measurements before you buy. Machines can vary greatly in size. For example, a leg-curl unit from one company may be 2 feet by 4 feet, whereas the same machine from another company may be 4 feet by 4 feet. Some multistation units require up to 250 square feet of floor space. Before you shop, measure how much floor space you have available; if space is tight, don't estimate.

With multigyms, it's crucial to try every station/exercise before buying. While doing so, ask yourself the following questions: Do the cables, weightstraps, or levers move smoothly and quietly? Am I comfortable in each position I'll employ during my workout? Are the seats and pads comfortable and easy to adjust? Make sure the padding on seats and armrests is adequate; foam that's too thin will not be comfortable. And make sure the padding is well-secured; watch out for cheap stapling or stitching.

# WEIGHT STACK EXERCISES

Today's multistation units typically offer the following stations: chest press, shoulder press, leg extension, prone or standing leg curl, triceps extension, triceps pushdown, arm curl, low rowing, lat pulldown, pec deck fly, upright rowing, and heel raise. Numerous other exercises can be performed. The particular exercises in this chapter are being demonstrated on a Schwinn® Home Trainer 730 multistation machine. Execution of a specific exercise may vary depending on the type of machine used.

# PEC DECK FLY

**Starting Position:** From the seated position, place your elbows or upper arms against the bottom of the pads. Keep your triceps parallel with the floor.

**Movement:** Bring your elbows together so the pads touch in front. Slowly return to the starting position. Maintain only a light grip on

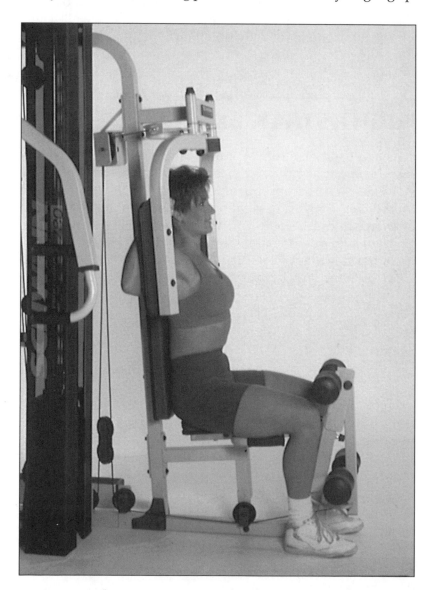

## PEC DECK FLY

the top of the pads, allowing your chest muscles to perform the work.

**Muscles Emphasized:** Pectorals; this exercise isolates the pectoral region more than does the chest press.

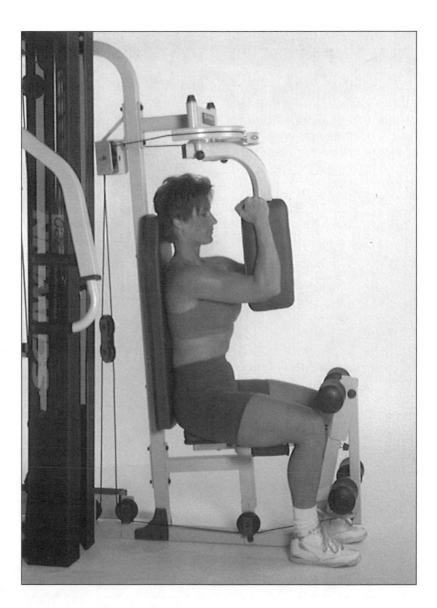

## CHEST PRESS

**Starting Position:** Seated in the vertical chest position, adjust the seat using the pop pin so that the handles are positioned even with the lower portion of the chest.

**Movement:** From the seated position, grip the handles and push forward by extending your elbows. Keep your shoulders and hips in place, and do not arch your lower back.

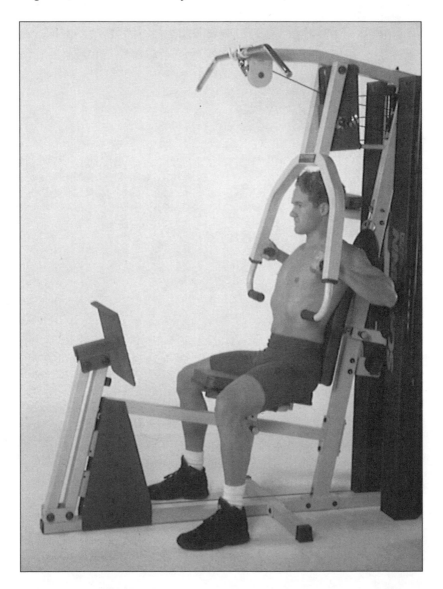

## CHEST PRESS

**Muscles Emphasized:** Deltoids, triceps, and pectorals; helps strengthen the muscles of the chest and front of shoulders.

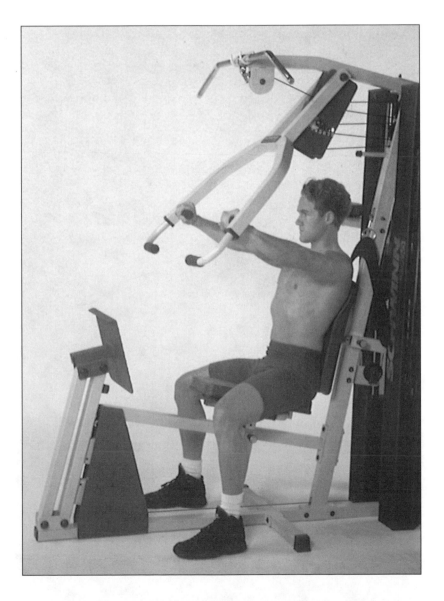

# TRICEPS EXTENSION

**Starting Position:** Seated on the chest press station, reach overhead and grasp the abdominal strap with both hands, palms facing upward. Lean forward until your torso is at a 45-degree angle. Your elbows should be bent, your upper arms should be aligned with your ears, your lower arms should be back, and there should be tension on the cable.

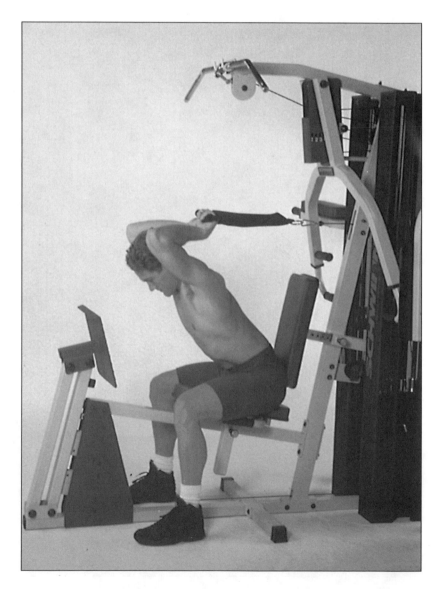

## TRICEPS EXTENSION

**Movement:** Keeping your upper arms stationary, push                  arms out until your elbows are straight. Hold briefly. Breathe out when pushing your arms out and breathe in when returning to the starting position.

**Muscles Emphasized:** Triceps; firms and strengthens the back of the upper arm.

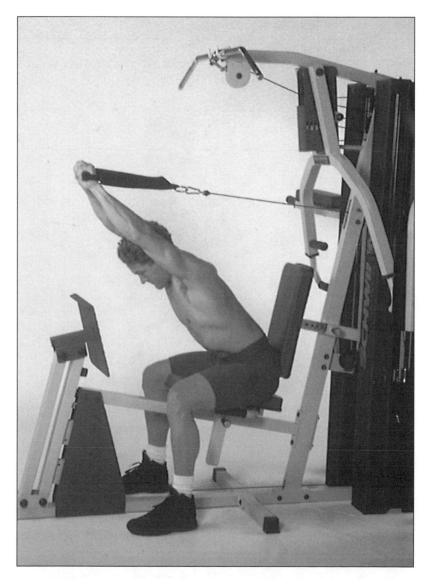

# TRICEPS PUSHDOWN

**Starting Position:** Stand facing the upper pulley station. Grasp the bar with both palms facing the floor. Your upper arms should be held stationary, and your lower arms should be bent at a 45-degree angle. Be sure to bend your knees, keep your torso erect, and relax your head and neck.

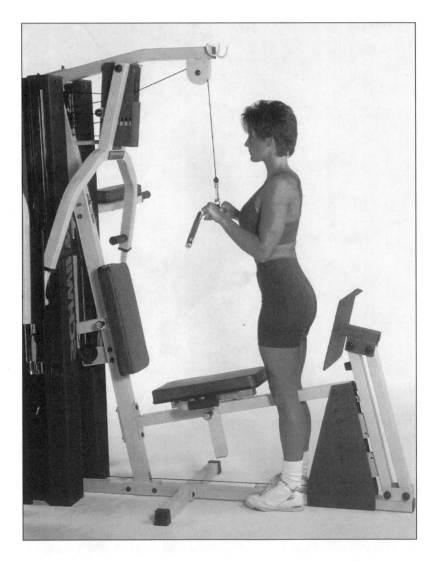

## TRICEPS PUSHDOWN

**Movement:** Place your hands about 3 inches apart with palms facing downward. Straighten your elbow joints until your arms are straight, keeping your elbows alongside your torso throughout entire movement. Slowly return to the starting position (elbows fully bent).

**Muscles Emphasized:** Triceps; this is the best exercise for developing and firming the back of the arm.

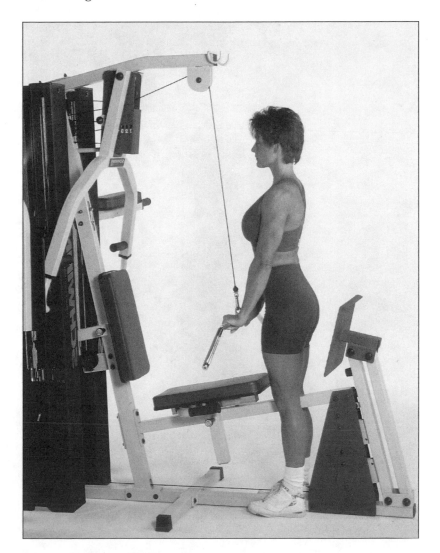

# SHOULDER PRESS

**Starting Position:** Seated on the vertical bench station, adjust the seat using the pop pin until the handles are even with your chest. Grasp both handles with both palms facing the floor; lean forward, keeping your back straight until your torso is at a 45-degree angle to the floor. Keep your feet flat on the floor.

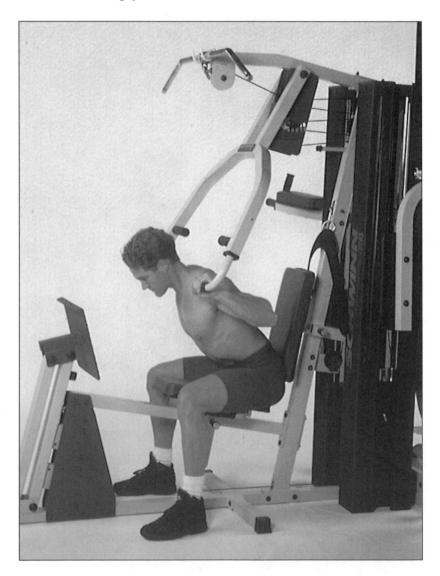

# SHOULDER PRESS

**Movement:** Press the handles straight up, away from your torso. Be sure to breathe out on the push and breathe in on the return to the starting position.

**Muscles Emphasized:** Deltoids; strengthens the muscles of the shoulder.

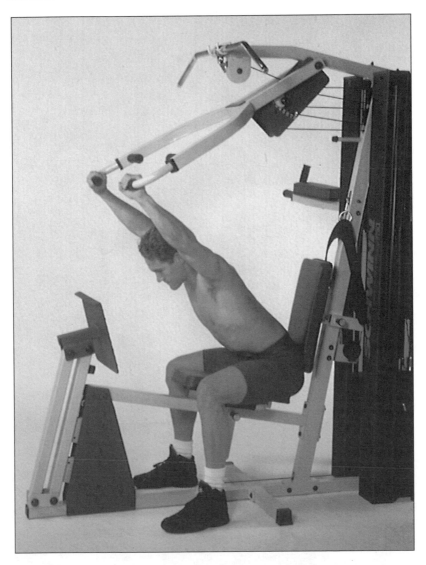

## LAT PULLDOWN

**Starting Position:** Seated on the vertical press station, under the overhead lat pulldown bar, grasp both handles, palms facing away from your body. The wider the grip, the more the isolation on the latissimus muscle. The narrower the grip, the more involvement the rhomboid muscles will have. Keep your feet flat on the floor and your head and neck relaxed.

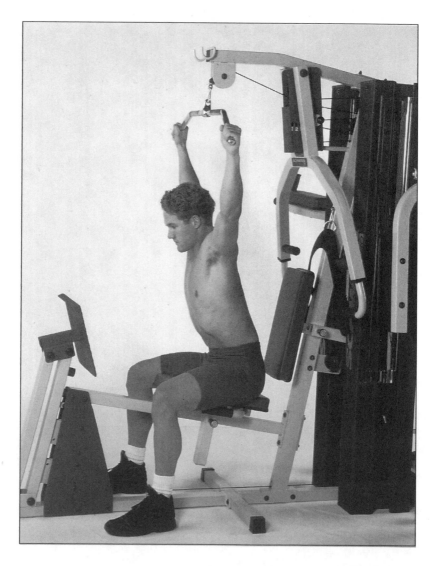

## LAT PULLDOWN

**Movement:** Pull your hands down from the overhead position. Keep your elbows wide and your hands behind your head. Contract your leg and abdominal muscles for stabilization. Breathe out when pulling the handles toward your shoulders, and breathe in when returning to the starting position.

**Muscles Emphasized:** Biceps, latissimus dorsi (large muscles of the upper back), and rhomboids.

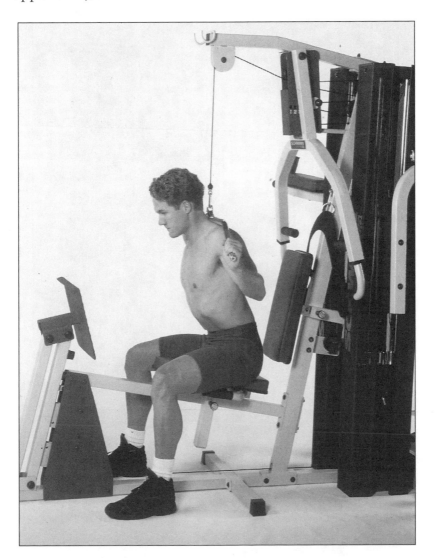

# UPRIGHT ROWING

**Starting Position:** Stand facing the low pulley station. Grasp the handle with your palms facing your body. Stand straight with your back erect, knees slightly bent, and head and neck relaxed.

**Movement:** Pull your hands up toward your shoulders, keeping your elbows wide so that your upper arms are horizontal and in line with your shoulders. At the peak position, your upper back

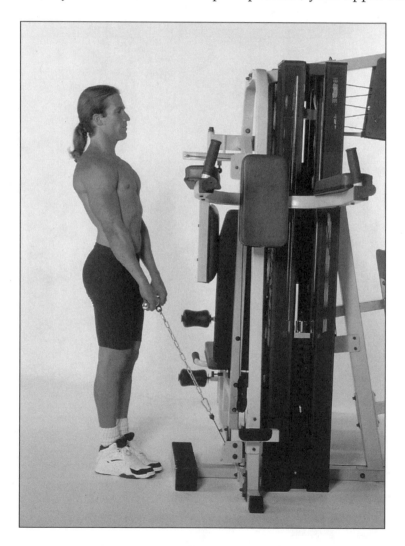

# UPRIGHT ROWING

and shoulder muscles must be completely contracted. Always maintain a straight trunk and neck. Be sure to keep your knees bent, and breathe in when pulling up and breathe out when returning to the starting position.

**Muscles Emphasized:** Trapezius, deltoids, and biceps—primarily muscles of the shoulder group.

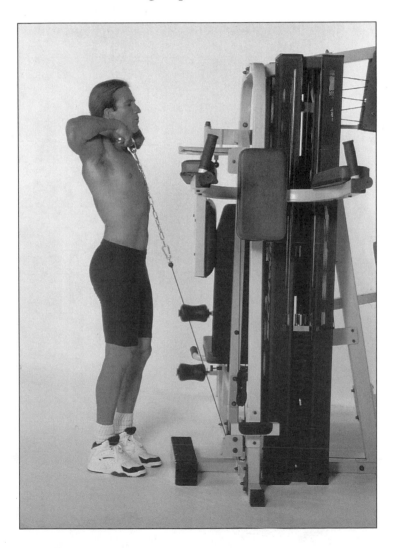

# LOW ROWING

**Starting Position:** Seated facing the lower pulley station, place your feet firmly against the machine. Grasp the handle with palms facing the floor. Sit back until your knees are only slightly bent; your heels should maintain a firm, stable position against the machine. Lean forward slightly about 10-15 degrees.

**Movement:** Draw your arms toward your lower chest. Be sure to keep your palms facing downward. Bend slightly at the waist, and only at the waist, when returning to the starting position. This

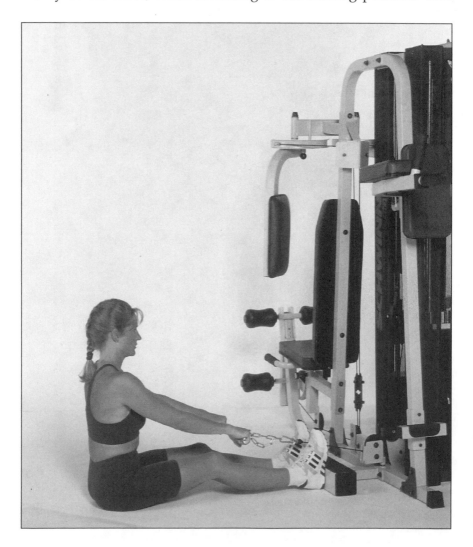

## LOW ROWING

allows for greater range of motion and greater isolation of the latissimus muscle. Caution: Do not lean your upper body back beyond a perpendicular, erect position when pulling the handles toward your chest.

**Muscles Emphasized:** Latissimus dorsi, biceps brachii, and spinal erectors; this exercise is designed to strengthen and stretch the upper, middle, and lower back as well as the extensor muscles of the shoulder joint.

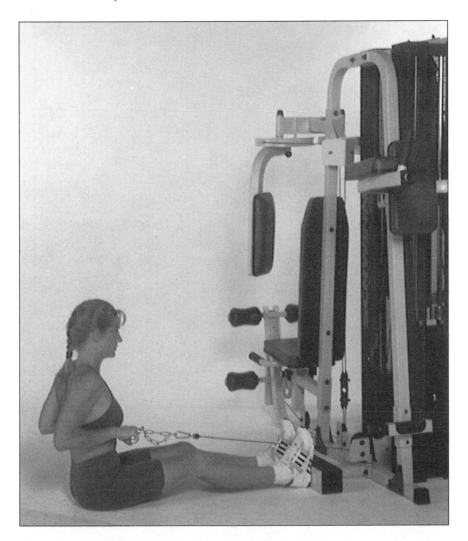

## ARM CURL

**Starting Position:** Stand facing the low pulley station of the machine, and grasp the bar with both hands facing forward. Bend your knees slightly. Your torso should be erect, and your head and neck should be relaxed.

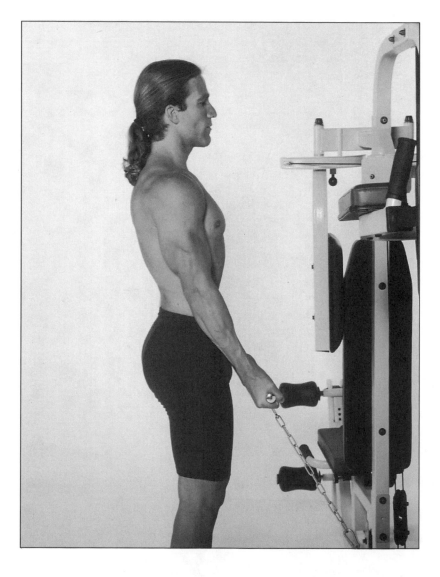

## ARM CURL

**Movement:** Bending at the elbow only, slowly curl your forearms toward your upper arms, keeping your upper arms stationary. Breathe out when curling your forearms up, and breathe in when returning to the starting position.

**Muscles Emphasized:** Biceps and forearm flexors; this is a popular exercise for isolating and developing the biceps (upper arm) for strength development.

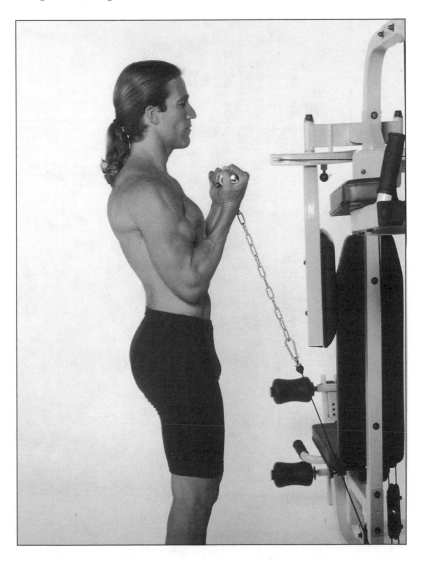

## HEEL RAISE

**Starting Position:** Stand in front of the low pulley station. Step into the heel raise belt and stand with the balls of your feet on the block. Your heels will drop below the block, and you should stand upright with your knees bent, head and back straight, and hands holding the frame of the machine.

**Movement:** Raise up on your toes until your heels are above the balls of your feet or you're standing on your tiptoes. As you return to the

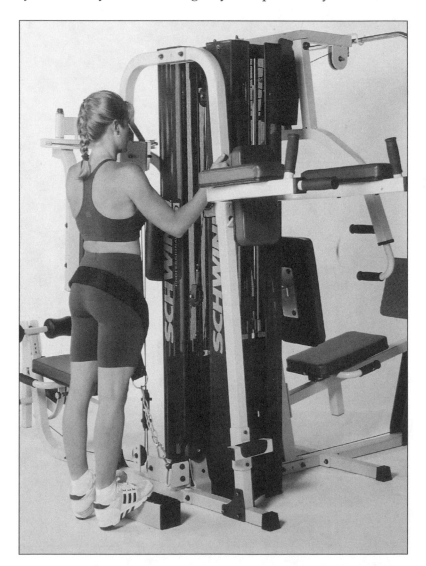

# HEEL RAISE

starting position, allow your heels to drop below the platform. This will allow you to achieve a full range of motion. Remember to breathe normally.

**Muscles Emphasized:** Gastrocnemius and soleus; this exercise helps develop the calf muscles while building power and endurance in the lower legs; it may also increase ankle range of motion.

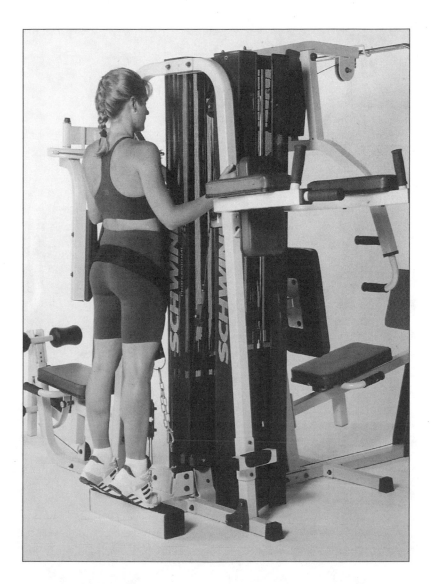

## LEG EXTENSION

**Starting Position:** Using the leg extension station, adjust the seat until your knees and hips are in alignment and your legs are parallel to the floor. The lower pads should rest slightly above your feet on the front of your ankles.

**Movement:** Extend your feet straight out and away from the machine, moving slowly until your legs are straight but not hyperextended. Hold this position for 1 second, then slowly return to the

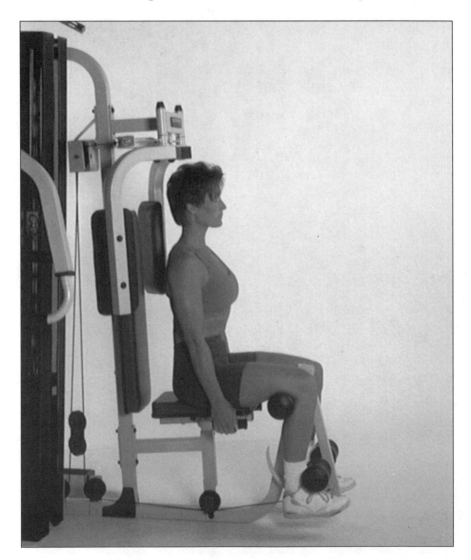

# LEG EXTENSION

starting position. Remember to always move with controlled speed. Breathe out when extending your legs, and breathe in when returning to the starting position.

**Muscles Emphasized:** Quadriceps (rectus femoris, vastus medialis, and vastus lateralis); this exercise allows you to isolate the muscles of the front of the thigh while developing strength and stability in the muscles that surround the knee.

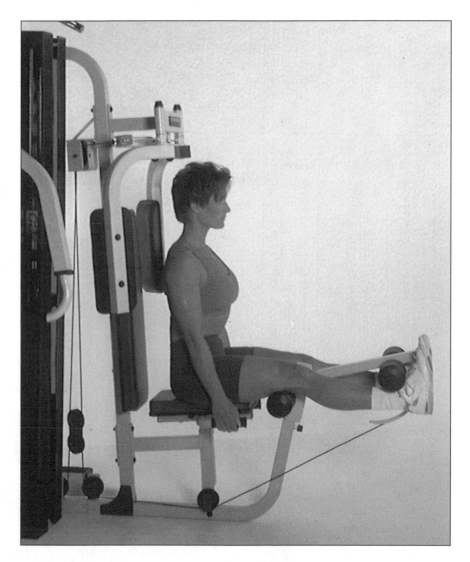

## STANDING LEG CURL

**Starting Position:** Stand facing the machine on either side of the leg extension station. Using the pop pin, adjust the knee pad to a height slightly above your knee. Stand straight with your support leg slightly bent and your head and neck relaxed. Reach out and grasp the machine for support.

**Movement:** Moving only at the knee, bend your knee and bring your heel as close to the rear as possible. Remember to move in a

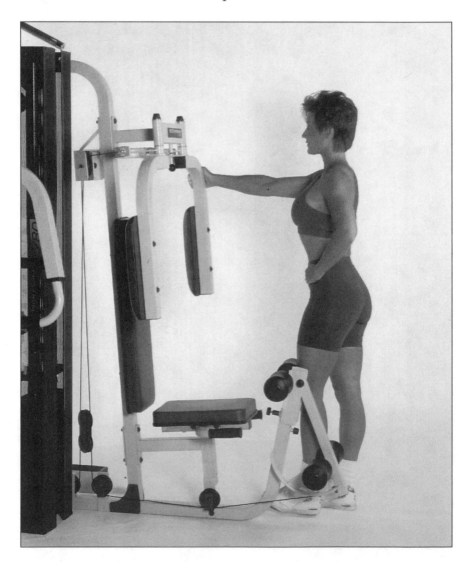

## STANDING LEG CURL

controlled manner and extend your leg as straight as possible when returning to the starting position. Breathe out when curling your leg up, and breathe in when returning to the starting position.

**Muscles Emphasized:** Hamstrings (biceps femoris, semitendinosus, and semimembranosus); these are the primary muscles involved in propelling the body forward when walking or running.

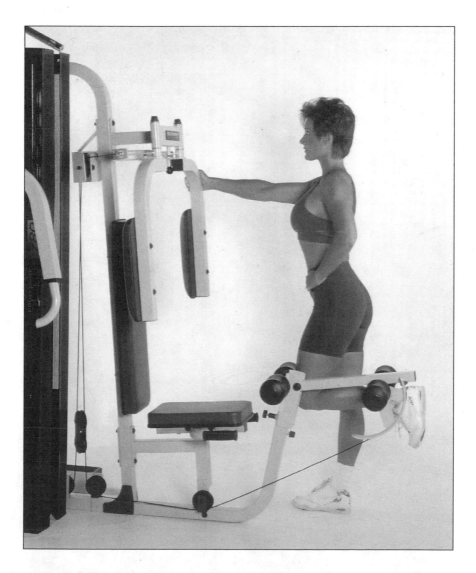

# ABDOMINAL CRUNCHES

**Starting Position:** While seated in the vertical press station, use the pop pin to lower the seat and adjust the back support so that your shoulders are below the abdominal pulley station. Adjust the back support out far enough so that when pulling on the straps, there is a prestress on the cable. Reach overhead and grasp the abdominal crunch straps, drawing them toward your body, pulling them over your shoulder. Keep your palms facing inward, your back erect, and your feet flat on the floor. If your machine does not have this station, perform this exercise on the floor.

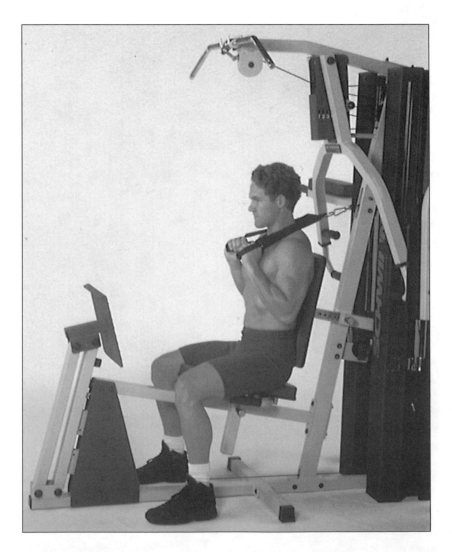

# ABDOMINAL CRUNCHES

**Movement:** While keeping your feet firmly planted on the floor, curl your torso toward your knees. Remember to pull from your stomach (abdominal) area and not your upper body. Breathe out when pulling toward your knees, and breathe in when returning to the starting position.

**Muscles Emphasized:** Rectus abdominis (stomach muscles).

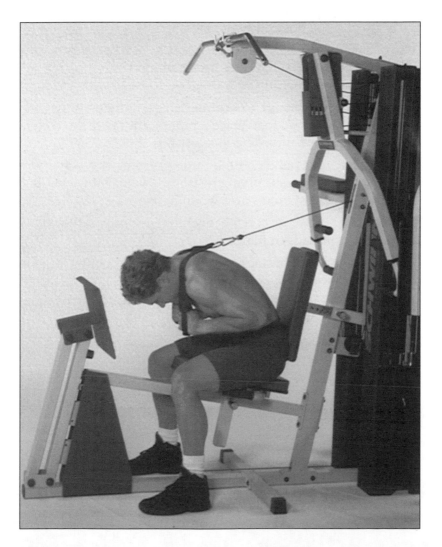

## ✓ INJURY PREVENTION

Before progressing to a heavier weight, be sure that you are ready to lift more. Increasing weights too soon can cause your technique to suffer and may lead to injury.

Keep your mind on what you are doing. Concentrate while you are performing an exercise, and pay especially close attention when you are changing plates or setting loads.

Do not hold your breath during exertion. Slowly exhale during the exertion phase and inhale during the recovery phase. Holding your breath may result in a Valsalva maneuver in which blood flow is temporarily cut off, resulting in higher blood pressure and the possibility of blacking out.

Use of a weightlifting belt is optional. Use of a belt is generally overrated and does not reduce the likelihood of injury. If a belt is used, keep it snug during lifting and loose between sets.

Check your equipment (machine cables, pulleys, pins) frequently for wear and tear. Once a month, lubricate the weight stack guide rods with a dry silicon spray.

Never place your hands on the pulley system or reach under lifted plates that are supplying resistance. Check the lever that locks an exercise station's arm when in use.

Place your hands or feet on the machine carefully so they don't slip off the roll pads or handles.

Don't drop the weight stack at the end of each repetition; lower it gently to its starting point.

If possible, strength train with another person for spotting purposes.

# CLOSING SET

In the 45 years since Universal Gym introduced the first multistation weight machine in the 1950s, the multistation gym has become the staple of home strength-conditioning equipment. Today, although many fitness enthusiasts are turning to free weights, the multistation machine is holding its own in the home fitness market.

Multistation machines still possess advantages unmatched by any other type of exercise machine, and they continue to provide a space- and cost-efficient method of training.

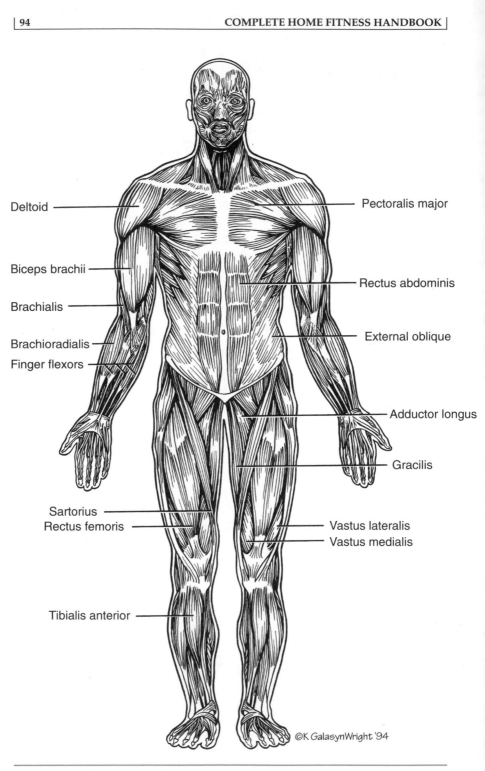

Deltoid

Biceps brachii

Brachialis

Brachioradialis

Finger flexors

Sartorius
Rectus femoris

Tibialis anterior

Pectoralis major

Rectus abdominis

External oblique

Adductor longus

Gracilis

Vastus lateralis
Vastus medialis

©K GalasynWright '94

Front view of human muscles.
© K. Galasyn-Wright, Champaign, IL, 1994.

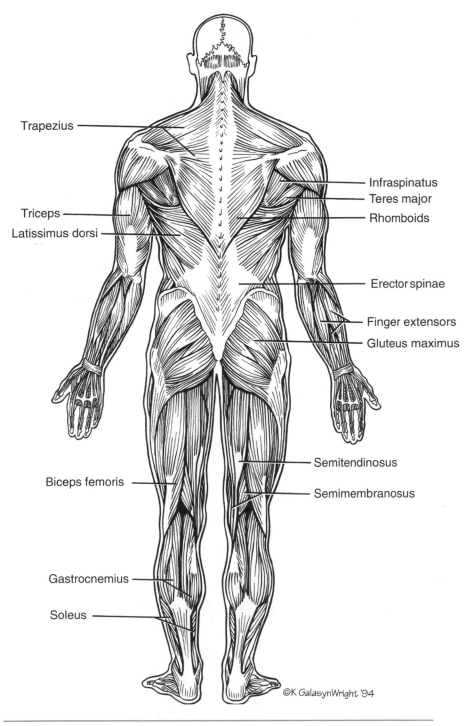

Rear view of human muscles.
© K. Galasyn-Wright, Champaign, IL, 1994.

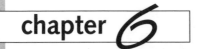

chapter 6

# Lifting Free Weights

### Harvey S. Newton, MA, CSCS

*I*n the days before resistance training machines were invented, all weight training was done using what we now call "free weights." This recent addition to our vocabulary came about as a means of differentiating between exercising on a machine and using the old standbys, barbells and dumbbells.

For the average person setting up a home gym, free weights provide excellent strength training benefits. They easily complement home fitness equipment and make it possible to do a complete selection of exercises in the privacy of a house or an apartment. You'll enjoy the variety, but it's important to know what you're getting into and what lies ahead. Let's take a look at some of the basics.

## WHAT DO I NEED?

The free weight equipment needed to strength train at home consists simply of barbells and dumbbells, both of which can be purchased fairly inexpensively at most sporting goods or fitness equipment stores. For those on a tight budget, these items are frequently found at used sporting equipment stores and garage sales. The complete home gym should have both barbell and dumbbell capabilities.

Barbells are long, solid bars with removable weight plates on each end. Two types of barbells are available: the exercise bar, usually 1-1/8 inches in diameter throughout its length, and the Olympic-standard bar, with about the same diameter bar but with an outside sleeve (where the plates slide on and off) diameter of about 2 inches. Plates of various weights are available, and these are placed on each end of the bar. Always be sure to fix the bar's collars, or locking clips, securely in place to avoid unexpected shifting of the plates.

Dumbbells are short, solid bars that are held in each hand. They come either with adjustable weight plates on each end or in a one-piece configuration with nonadjustable weight on the ends. Dumb-bell bars are normally about 12 inches long and 1-1/8 inches in diameter. You only need one pair of adjustable dumbbells along with plenty of plates to provide the proper resistance for different exercises. If you use one-piece dumbbells, you will need several pairs of different weights. Of course, the advantage of one-piece dumbbells is that the weights cannot fall off the ends.

Barbells are appropriate for exercises that require heavy weights. However, because both hands are lifting the same object, muscle imbalance, such as when one arm is weaker than the other, may go untreated. Many exercises call for barbells to be placed on the shoulders or upper back. This can make it difficult to get rid of the weight quickly and safely, if necessary, as in loss of balance.

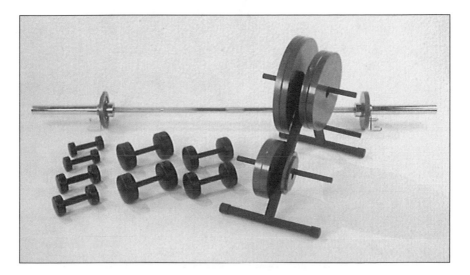

Because dumbbells are held singly in each hand, less weight is used for the same exercise than would be used with a barbell. The arms and hands must constantly hold the weights, which can cause fatigue; however, if you need to drop the weights quickly for any reason, it is much easier and safer to do so with dumbbells.

## ADDITIONAL EQUIPMENT CONSIDERATIONS

In addition to a multipurpose resistance training machine and free weight equipment, only one or two other items are needed to create a workout area that will allow you to work every muscle group completely. After the purchase of weights, the most important pieces

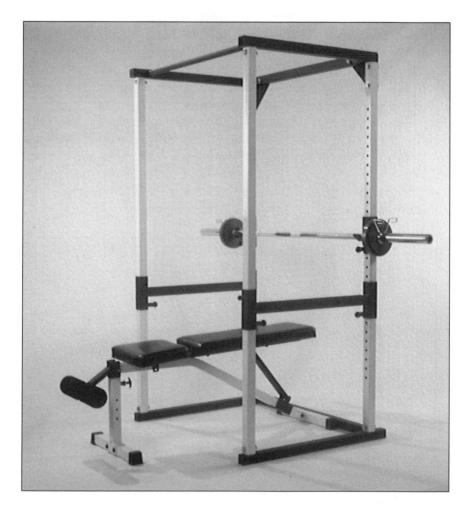

of equipment are a bench and a set of squat racks. There are many inexpensive benches on the market; check the quality carefully if you expect to employ heavy weights in exercises such as the bench press. Make sure the width and thickness of the bench pad are adequate, as performing a bench press with a narrow, thin pad can lead to bruising around the shoulder blades, not to mention discomfort.

Squat racks come in varying styles, with the simplest consisting of two adjustable uprights with a yoke top to hold a barbell securely until you lift it off the standards. The bases need to be wide enough (round or square) to support the weight of the barbell, even if you drop it heavily back into place. Squat racks come in handy for any exercise in which you want to lift the bar from an elevated starting position rather than having to pick it up from the floor. This would include overhead pressing motions and most leg exercises such as squats or lunges. An enclosed power rack (pictured on p. 98) with adjustable bars that will hold the barbell if you cannot fully rise from a squat can add safety in the home gym.

## WHAT TO WEAR

Weightlifting belts are popular with many people, but they are not necessary. For overhead movements or lifts with the barbell on the

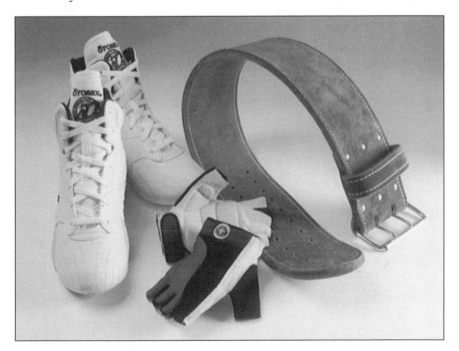

shoulders, such as the squat, a belt can provide some support to the lower back by allowing for increased intra-abdominal pressure. However, belts serve little purpose for most other exercises, including those done lying down or seated. Even if you're squatting, it is generally recommended that you lift several light sets without the belt to develop the supporting muscles around the abdominal wall. The belt may then be used for the heaviest weights. Don't be fooled into thinking a belt will keep you from becoming injured—it won't.

Gloves are also popular for weight lifting. They can help eliminate callous development, but they are certainly not a necessary part of lifting garb.

Shoes should be a solid court or cross-training model with a rubber sole, without flared heels. Many running shoes are not well suited for weight training, so don't just grab the first pair of sport shoes in your closet.

# PROS AND CONS OF FREE WEIGHTS

A long-standing argument in the field of strength training centers around the question, Which is better for me, free weights or machines? There is no simple answer, as both have benefits and disadvantages. Most training programs are enhanced by using exercises in both the free weight and the machine categories; however, if you're thinking of outfitting your home gym with only free weights, let's examine both sides of the issue.

There are several advantages to free weights.

- Cost—One of the primary benefits of using free weights in the home gym is the low cost of this type of equipment.

- Large variety of movements—You can move free weights in any direction the human body can go. This becomes particularly important when developing a muscle through a variety of movements rather than being stuck in just one plane of movement.

- Training of skill-related movements—Balance is certainly enhanced during free weight exercises in which you are not seated. This cannot be said for resistance machines. In some sports, specific speed of movement is required. This can be more easily trained with free weights than with most machines.

- Space considerations—Free weights take up very little space compared to most machines, which can be a benefit in limited quarters.

- Safety—Many people's first impression is that free weights are more dangerous than machines. Actually, recent safety statistics have shown resistance training machines to have a slightly higher incidence of injuries, but this will remain a point of contention for some time. If you don't have strength training experience, machines may be a safer way to start.

There are also a few drawbacks to free weights.

- Instruction—Unlike machines, use of free weights may require guidance from an experienced instructor. The National Strength and Conditioning Association certifies both Certified Strength and Conditioning Specialists and Certified Personal Trainers. A qualified instructor can check to make sure that your technique is correct, or that you're not cheating to lift more than you can properly lift in strict style.

- Clutter—Weights tend to get scattered around, which can lead to losing plates, slipping on weights inadvertently left around, and so on. These problems won't happen with a machine.

- Noise—Free weights make a clatter when putting plates on the bar. Weights are also sometimes dropped due to either the weight involved, a failed lift, or carelessness. This can be very annoying to those living in an apartment below you!

# BASIC EXERCISES

As mentioned earlier, there are hundreds of exercises that can be performed with free weights. In this chapter, we'll concentrate on the basics. Most other movements are simply variations of these.

It makes sense to divide your workout into four segments: (a) lower body, (b) torso (low back and abdominal), (c) upper body pushing, and (d) upper body pulling. Starting with the lower body, exercises should include movements for the calves, quadriceps, hamstrings, and hips. Pushing or pulling movements can be either single- or multiple-joint exercises. If time is a concern, use a multiple-joint lift that works several muscle groups at the same time. If you have the time, single-joint movements can be added to the workout for further muscle development. Strive to create a balanced training program. Address your weaknesses as well as your strengths.

Always warm up for 5 to 10 minutes prior to weight training. Warming up raises the body's core temperature and prepares the muscles for work. It is a good idea to follow each workout with a cool-down period of similar length. Cool-down includes stretching and light movements to eliminate waste products from the muscles.

## BACK EXTENSION

**Starting Position:** Place a towel or pad under your hips while lying on the floor on your chest. Your hands should be alongside your hips.

**Movement:** Raise your shoulders and chest off the ground by contracting the muscles of your lower back.

**Muscles Emphasized:** Spinal erectors.

**Variations:** Holding your hands behind your head will add resistance to the exercise. After several weeks or months of performing this exercise, you may wish to do the full-range-of-motion back extension. This requires an elevated padded bench so that your feet and hips are supported while you bend forward approximately 90 degrees. Lift your torso to a position parallel to the floor. Important: Be sure your ankles are held securely by the bench or a spotter.

Perform the low row exercise on your home resistance training machine. Keeping your lower back straight (flat); begin with your torso inclined slightly forward. Pull your torso back until it is perpendicular to the floor, and pull the handles the rest of the way to your lower chest/abdomen area by bending your elbows.

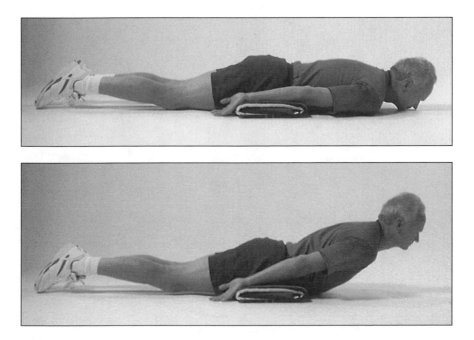

# HEEL RAISE

**Starting Position:** Take a barbell from the squat racks and rest it on your upper back (the trapezius muscles). Don't rest the bar on a vertebra. Step forward several feet and place your toes on a 2- by 4-inch board approximately 20 inches long.

**Movement:** Starting with your heels on the floor and your toes on the board, slowly raise up onto your toes, then slowly lower to the starting position.

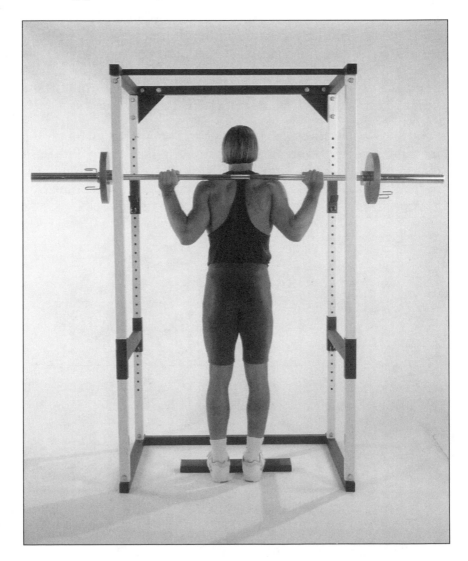

## HEEL RAISE

**Muscles Emphasized:** Lower leg (calf) muscles, primarily the gastrocnemius. Strengthening the calf muscles can be helpful to all sports in which the legs are key players (running, cycling, etc.).

**Variations:** Beginners should perform this movement with one foot at a time, holding a dumbbell in one hand (arm straight) and holding onto an object for balance with the other hand.

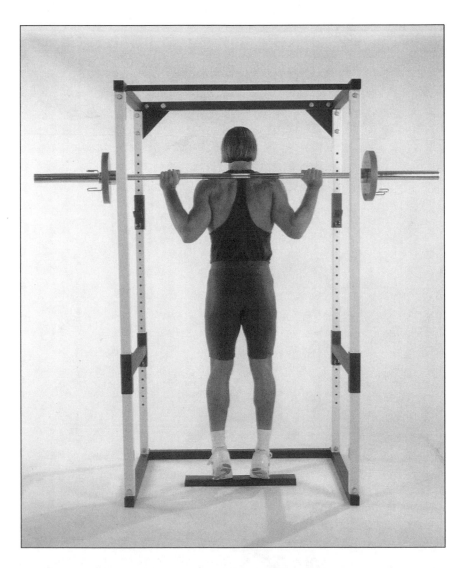

## SQUAT

**Starting Position:** Resting the bar on your upper back, lift the weights from the squat rack. Step back about 2 feet and assume a position with your feet flat on the floor, your toes pointed slightly outward, your back straight and flat, and your head in a neutral position with eyes straight ahead.

**Movement:** Slowly bend your ankles, knees, and hips, descending until the thighs are approximately parallel to the floor. Keep your feet flat, and keep any forward trunk incline to a minimum. Stand erect and repeat.

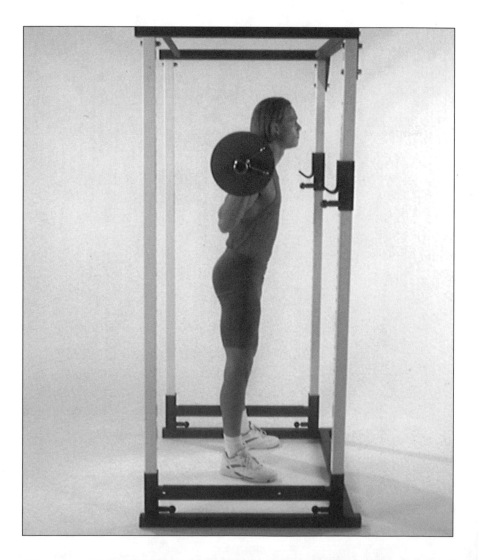

# SQUAT

**Muscles Emphasized:** Quadriceps, gluteus maximus, and spinal erectors. This movement greatly strengthens the lower body.

**Variations:** Dumbbells may be used, holding the weights either at the shoulders or at the junction of the hip and thigh (arms bend as the body descends).

*Note:* Don't be in a hurry to lift a lot of weight in the squat. In fact, for the first several workouts, you should practice the squat with only the weight of the empty bar so that you get the right balance. *Always use spotters for the squat exercise.*

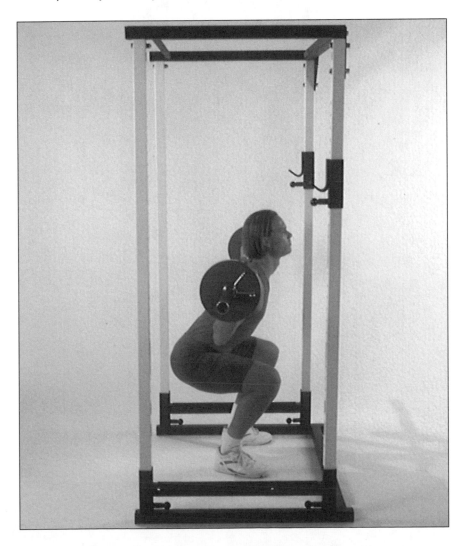

## LUNGE

**Starting Position:** Take the barbell from the squat racks as in the squat. Step back about 4 feet.

**Movement:** Step out about 30 inches with your right foot. The front foot should be absolutely flat and the rear foot should be supported on its toes. Bend your right knee until the thigh is about parallel to the floor. Keep the lower part of your right leg close to perpendicular to the floor. Push up and back with your right leg until your feet are in the starting position. Repeat with your left leg.

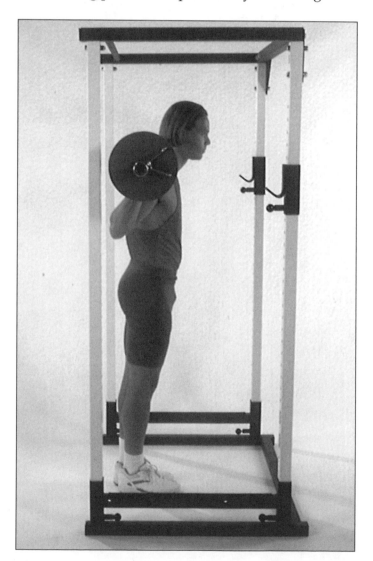

# LUNGE

**Muscles Emphasized:** Gluteus maximus, hamstrings, and quadriceps.

**Variations:** Perform all repetitions on one leg, then switch legs. Perform lunges with dumbbells instead of a barbell (arms straight, dumbbells at hips).

*Note:* Practicing this movement without weight is recommended.

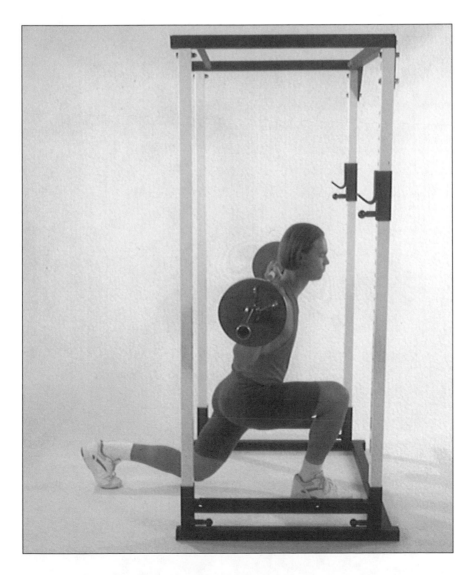

## GOOD MORNING

**Starting Position:** Place the bar on your upper back. A single dumb-bell can be used, but a towel or other padding will be necessary.

**Movement:** With your knees slightly bent, keep your back absolutely flat and bend forward at the waist until your back is nearly parallel to the floor. At no time allow your back to round. Recover slowly to the starting position.

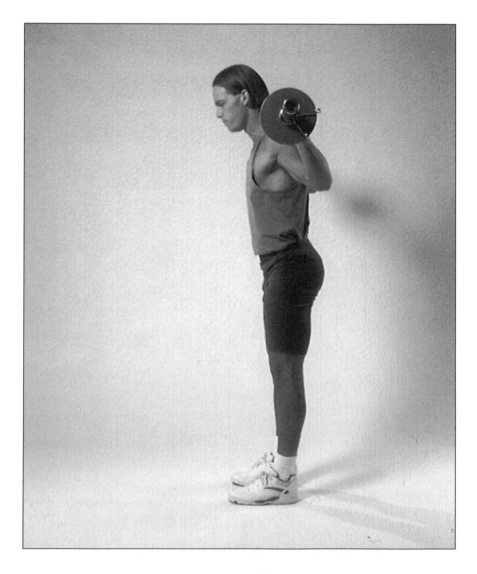

## GOOD MORNING

**Muscles Emphasized:** Hamstrings, spinal erectors.

*Note:* This is considered an advanced exercise and should not be attempted without adequate prior development of the lower back muscles and supervision. Beginners are advised to perform the leg curl exercise on their home resistance machine. Be conservative in performing this movement with weight. Use a light weight and work only with proper technique.

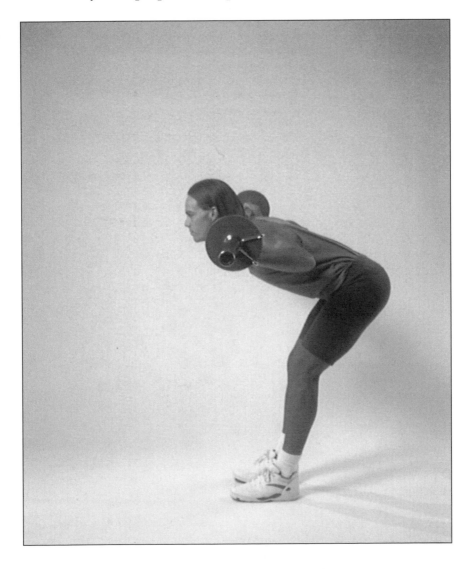

## STIFF-LEG DEAD LIFT

**Starting Position:** Pick up the barbell from the floor with a flat back, using your legs and hips to lift properly. Keep your back absolutely flat, your arms straight, and the barbell close to the centerline of your body. If dumbbells are used, hold them directly in front of your thighs, arms straight.

**Movement:** Slowly bend forward at the waist, lowering the bar to a position over your feet. Bend your knees slightly, keeping your back absolutely flat. Recover to a standing position.

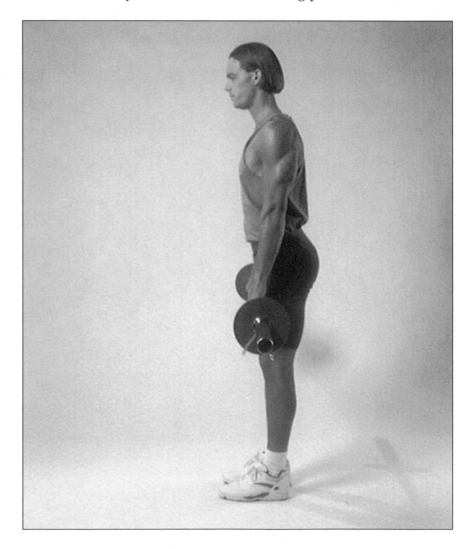

## STIFF-LEG DEAD LIFT

**Muscles Emphasized:** Hamstrings, spinal erectors.

**Variation:** If the barbell plates touch the floor easily, consider standing on a solid elevated surface that will allow the bar to be lowered further.

*Note:* This is considered an advanced exercise and should not be attempted without adequate prior development of the lower back muscles and supervision. Beginners are advised to perform the leg curl exercise on their home resistance machine. Be conservative in performing this movement with weight. Use a light weight and work only with proper technique.

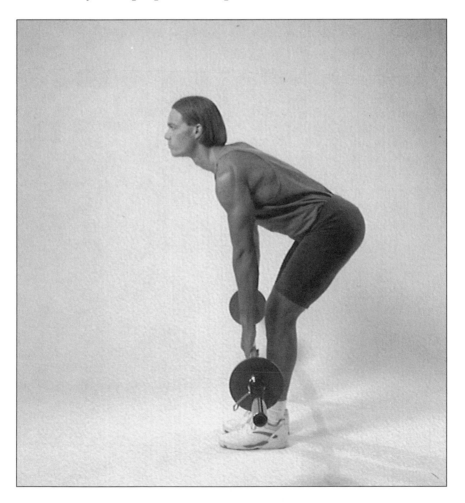

# BENCH PRESS

**Starting Position:** Lie flat on the bench with your feet flat on the floor and your hips and head flat on the bench. Use moderate hand spacing (knuckles facing you, palms facing the ceiling). Lift the barbell from the uprights and position it over your chest, arms straight.

**Movement:** Slowly lower the bar to your chest and then press straight up.

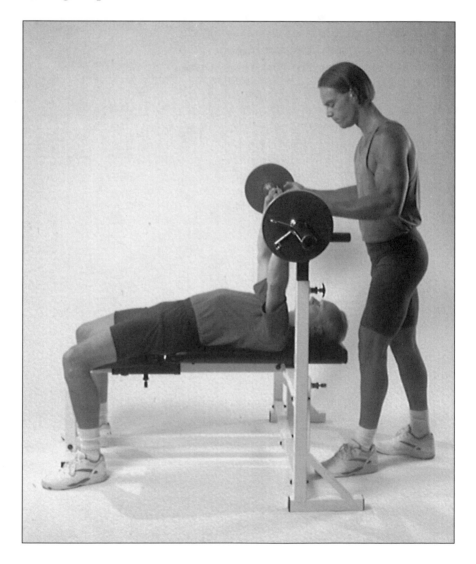

## BENCH PRESS

**Muscles Emphasized:** Pectorals (chest), deltoids (shoulders), and triceps (back of arms).

**Variation:** Pressing motion can be done with either a barbell or a pair of dumbbells. An incline or decline press can be performed, but a special bench is needed.

*Note:* Always use spotters for the bench press exercise.

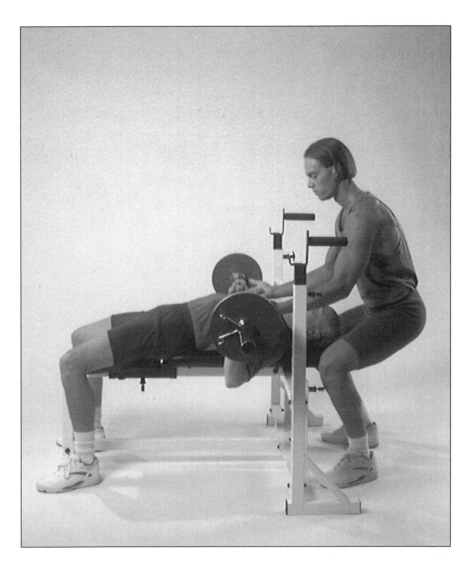

## SHOULDER PRESS

**Starting Position:** Lift the barbell either off the squat racks or from the floor so that the bar rests on your arms (which are fully bent) and is supported by your shoulders and clavicles.

**Movement:** While keeping your torso straight, press the barbell overhead until your elbows are straight.

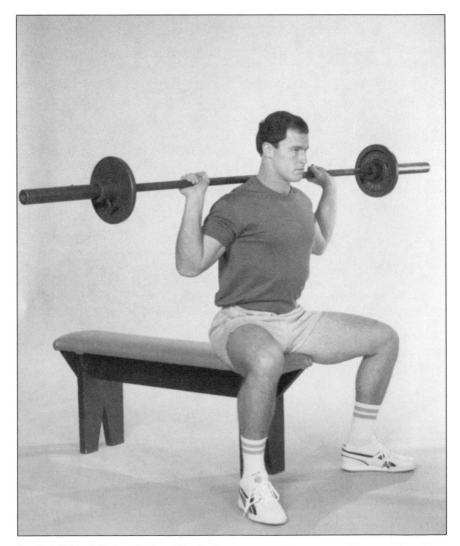

Seated behind-the-neck shoulder press.

# SHOULDER PRESS

**Muscles Emphasized:** Deltoids (shoulders) and triceps (back of arms).

**Variation:** The pressing motion can be done with either a barbell or a pair of dumbbells. The bar can be placed on the upper back and lifted behind the head (press behind neck). All pressing motions can be done while seated.

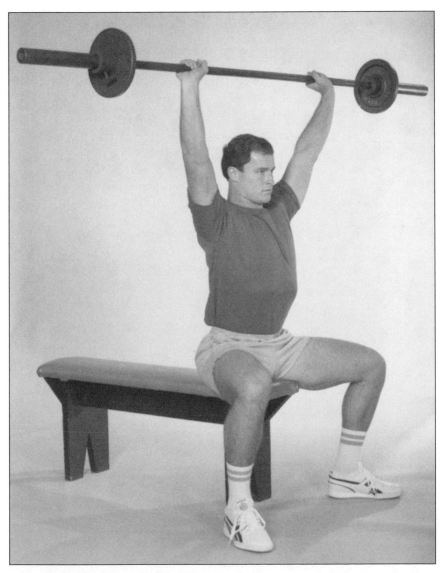

Seated behind-the-neck shoulder press.

# TRICEPS PRESS

**Starting Position:** Place weight overhead, palms facing up, arms straight. With a barbell, use a close grip and keep your elbows close to your head.

**Movement:** Lower weight to a position behind your neck. Press overhead.

**Muscles Emphasized:** Triceps (arm extensors).

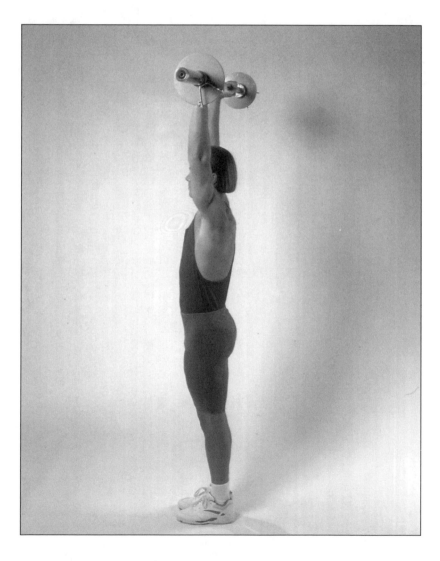

# TRICEPS PRESS

**Variations:** With a dumbbell, interlace the fingers of both hands to hold the dumbbell securely by its discs (hands inside). If you are using adjustable dumbbells, be sure the collars are fastened securely. This exercise can be performed while seated or while lying on your back on a bench and lowering the barbell behind your head.

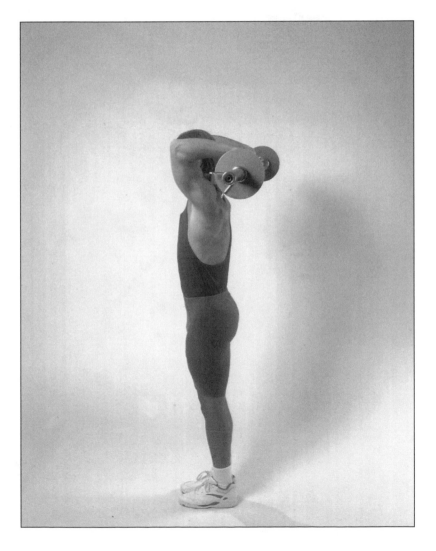

# TRICEPS KICKBACK

**Starting Position:** Hold a dumbbell in your left hand. Support your right knee and right hand on a flat bench. Bend at the waist, keeping your bent left elbow tucked in close to your side with the dumbbell pointed toward the floor.

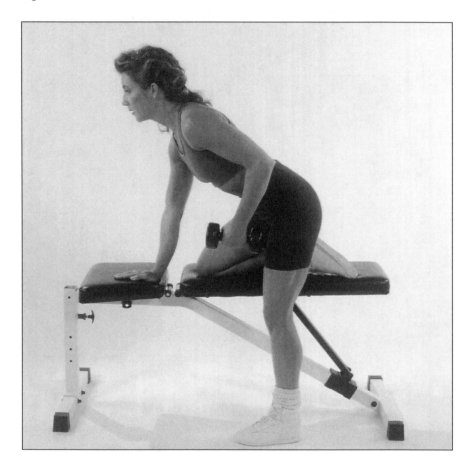

# TRICEPS KICKBACK

**Movement:** Slowly extend, or straighten, your elbow in a "kicking back" motion.

**Muscles Emphasized:** Triceps (arm extensors).

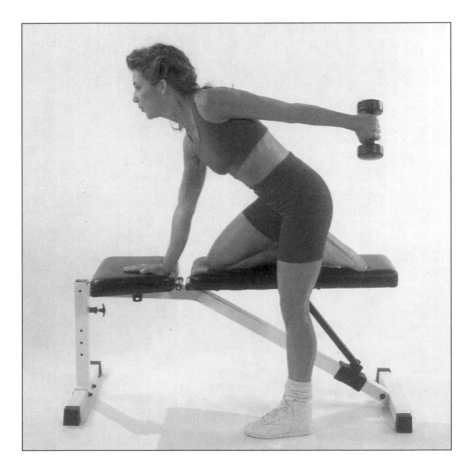

# BENT-OVER ROW

**Starting Position:** Stand holding a barbell. Bend at the waist until your torso is nearly parallel to the floor with your knees slightly bent. Your back should be flat and your arms straight.

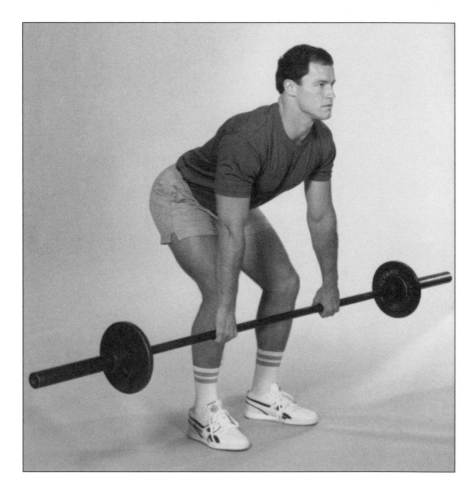

# BENT-OVER ROW

**Movement:** Pull the barbell smoothly up to your lower chest and return it to the starting position.

**Muscles Emphasized:** Latissimus dorsi, biceps.

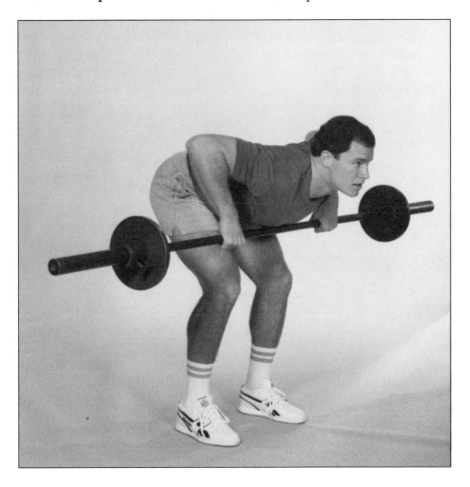

## ONE-ARM DUMBBELL ROW

**Starting Position:** Place the knee and hand of the nonpulling side on a bench. Bend over parallel to the floor with the dumbbell hanging straight down. Your back should be flat.

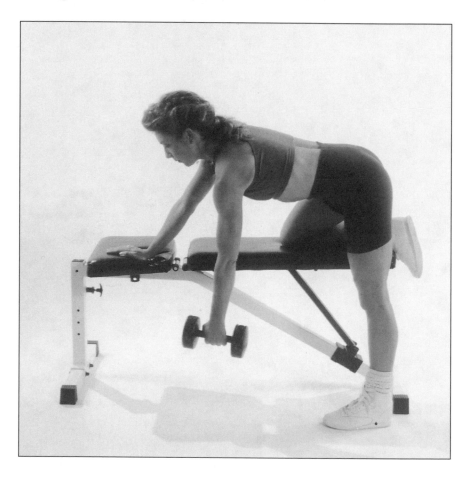

## ONE-ARM DUMBBELL ROW

**Movement:** Pull the weight up to your chest, then lower it to the starting position.

**Muscles Emphasized:** Latissimus dorsi, biceps.

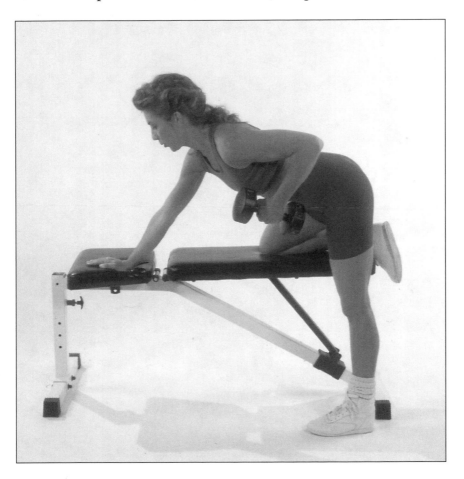

# UPRIGHT ROW

**Starting Position:** Stand with the bar resting at the top of your thighs, arms straight. Use an overhand grip with your hands about 4 to 6 inches apart.

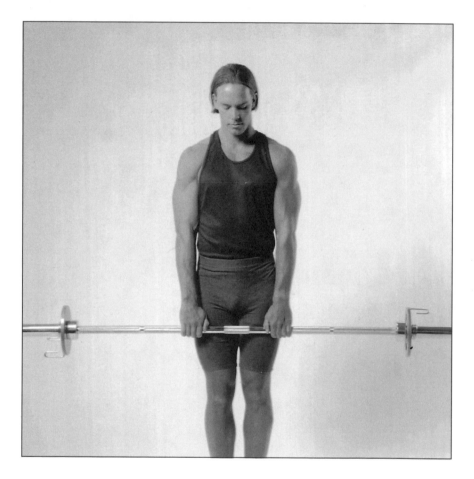

## UPRIGHT ROW

**Movement:** Bend your elbows to bring the barbell to a position just under your chin. Slowly lower the bar and repeat.

**Muscles Emphasized:** Trapezius, deltoids, biceps.

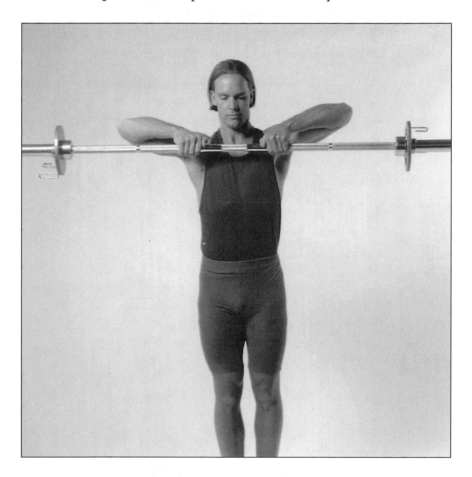

## ARM CURL

**Starting Position:** Stand erect holding a barbell or two dumbbells with an underhand grip.

**Movement:** Your elbows should be straight and held close to the sides of your body. Bend your elbows to raise the weight to a finishing position just under your chin.

**Muscles Emphasized:** Biceps and biceps brachii.

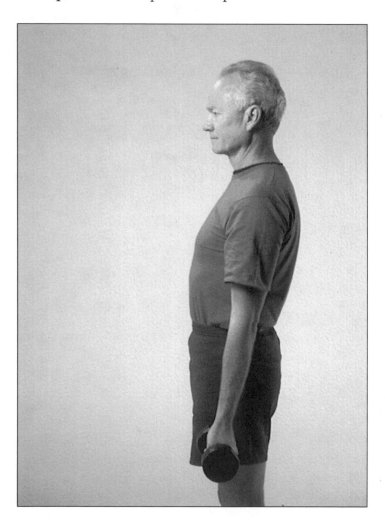

## ARM CURL

**Variations:** Perform the exercise while gripping the bar in an over-hand position (palms facing downward). This reverse curl places more emphasis on the forearm muscles. Dumbbells can be held in each hand and the curl performed by raising the dumbbells simultaneously or alternately. With dumbbells, the exercise can be performed while seated on a flat or inclined bench.

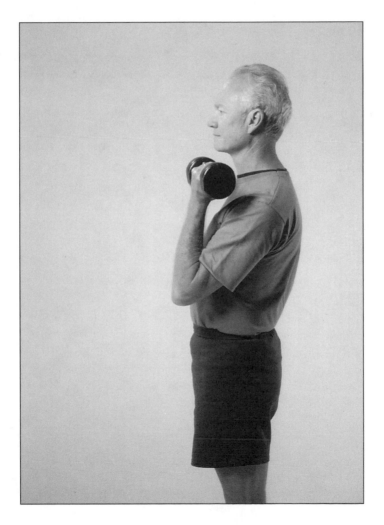

# FORWARD RAISE

**Starting Position:** Stand with a dumbbell in each hand, palms facing downward.

**Movement:** Raise one dumbbell in front of the body to about eye level (elbow slightly bent). As this weight is being lowered, begin

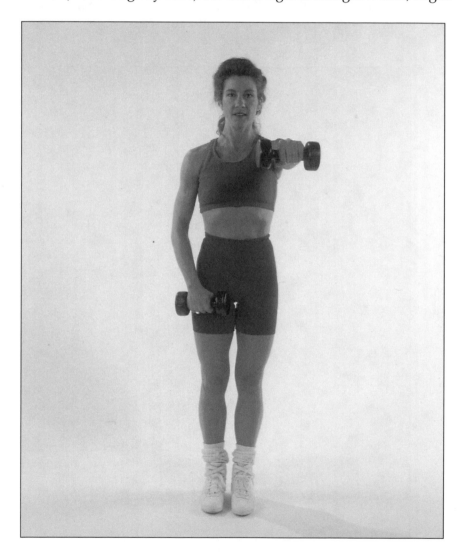

## FORWARD RAISE

raising the other dumbbell. Maintain a steady alternating motion for the desired number of repetitions.

**Muscles Emphasized:** Deltoids or shoulders, especially the front, or anterior, part.

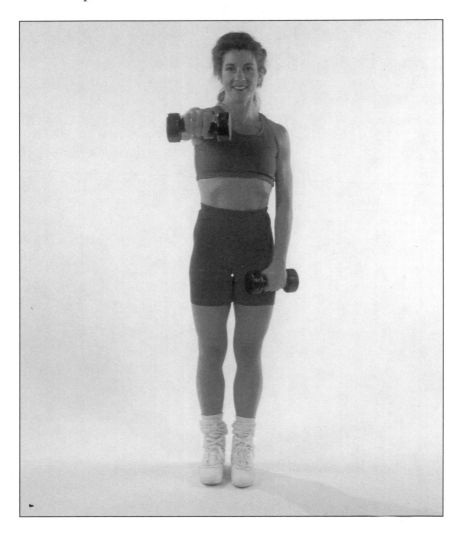

# LATERAL RAISE

**Starting Position:** Stand with a dumbbell in each hand, palms facing inward.

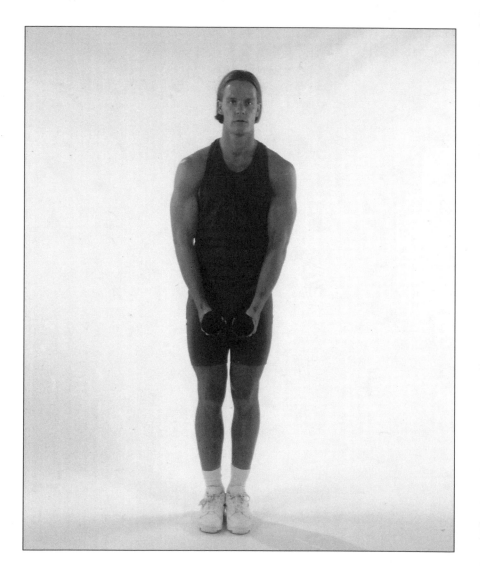

## LATERAL RAISE

**Movement:** Raise both dumbbells simultaneously to the side, stopping at about ear level. Lower to the starting position.

**Muscles Emphasized:** Deltoids, especially the lateral head.

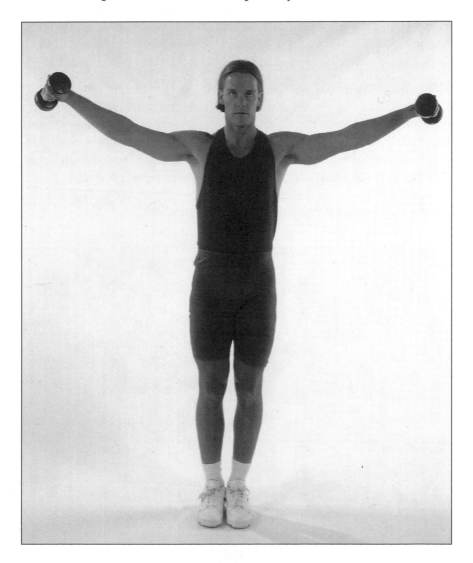

# TRUNK CURL

**Starting Position:** Lie on the floor with your knees bent and your feet and back flat on the floor. Your hands may be placed on the floor near your hips, across your chest, or behind your neck.

**Movement:** Curl your chin to your chest and raise your torso about 6 inches off the floor while keeping your lower back in contact with the floor.

**Muscles Emphasized:** Rectus abdominis.

**Variations:** Your feet can be placed on a bench about 18 inches high or they can simply be crossed and left free, with your hip joint at about a 90-degree bend. Attempt to raise yourself high enough to touch your elbows to your knees. Slowly lower and repeat. After you can do this 20 to 25 times with good form, place a small weight behind your head and continue to use resistance rather than aiming for an extremely high number of repetitions. This exercise can also be done on your home training unit.

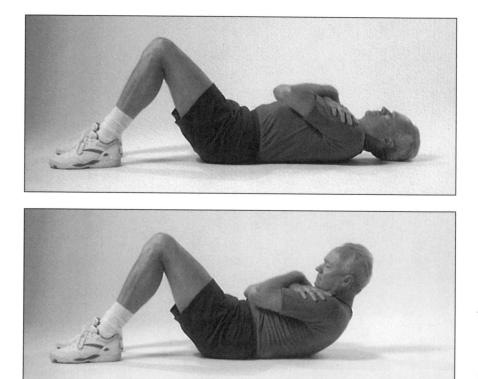

## ✓ INJURY PREVENTION

Be sure weights are loaded evenly on both sides.

Never lift free weights without collars securely locked in place.

Always use one or more spotters for the bench press and the squat.

Use spotters on any new exercise until you have developed the proper balance, especially with overhead lifts and in many dumbbell exercises.

Communicate with your spotter before getting in trouble.

If lifting from the floor, be sure to lift the weight safely with a flat back. Use your hips and legs to lift rather than your lower back.

Perform a movement through a complete range of motion. Do not use partial ranges of motion in order to lift heavier weight.

Start with the joint (elbow, for instance) completely open, then proceed to a closed joint.

Perform the movements at a steady pace. Do not allow gravity to take the weight quickly back to the starting position!

Take several seconds to execute the concentric (muscle-shortening) phase of the lift, followed by several seconds to lower the weight in the eccentric (muscle-lengthening) phase.

Stay tuned into what you are doing while lifting. Don't get distracted.

Exhale as you exert against the resistance. Inhale during the recovery portion of the exercise.

Don't hold your breath! If you have problems with elevated blood pressure, be especially careful not to hold your breath.

# FINAL THOUGHTS

There's no need to be intimidated by lifting free weights. Exercising with barbells and dumbbells is a challenging and fun activity that helps you develop additional strength, muscular endurance, and flexibility. The variety of movements available makes this an enjoyable experience, but be sure to learn the movements properly before attempting to lift heavier weights. Also keep in mind that to make continued improvements, you need to add weight in any exercise where the resistance seems to be getting easier.

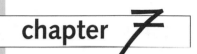

# chapter 7

# Riding Stationary Bikes

### Edmund R. Burke, PhD

*D*espite the variety of aerobic exercise equipment available for home gyms, stationary bicycles remain a constant in most homes. Cycling is undeniably a superb form of cardiovascular training, but doing it in the great outdoors is often counterproductive.

For one thing, without the aid of a heart rate monitor, it's impossible to check your pulse rate while riding outdoors. And have you ever tried keeping your heart rate at an aerobic level while weaving your road bicycle in and out of traffic? And those soaking rainstorms and bone-numbing cold snaps get old pretty fast.

The gap between the aerobic promise of cycling and the obstacles to doing it in the real world is one of the main reasons stationary cycling is (and has been for decades) the most popular indoor exercise. Another reason is that, in many ways, riding a stationary bicycle is superior to the real thing: The ride is smoother, the workout is more aerobically efficient, and the workout options are more varied. Best of all, you never get a flat tire on a stationary bicycle.

It hasn't always been that way. For years, stationary bicycles were seemingly designed by a deaf Marquis de Sade. They were uncomfortable, noisy, and made the exerciser feel as if they were exercising in a sauna due to the lack of airflow.

# COMPARING INDOOR BICYCLES

As the conventional bicycle celebrates its 150th birthday, its younger brother, the stationary bike, continues to be the number-one seller in home exercise equipment. But keeping abreast of the hundreds of makes and models of stationary bikes and the options available on them nowadays is about as easy as tracking the price of oil in the futures market.

The two most common types of home stationary bikes are brakepad and strap resistance. Brakepad bikes, which have a weighted fly-wheel and a system of brake calipers regulated by resistance—the control knob is usually located on or near the handlebars—are the lowest in cost. Strap-resistance bikes employ a nylon strap that tightens and loosens around a weighted flywheel. Although slightly more expensive than brakepad bikes, they generally ride smoother, have a wider range of resistance, and last longer.

An alternative to the strap-resistance and brakepad systems is the air-resistance bicycle. With these bikes, you get what you pay for (in the physical sense)—the harder you pedal, the more resistance you get. Air resistance bikes usually last longer because there is no friction involved in providing the resistance. These bikes also offer the consumer a cooling effect. As you pedal up a sweat, the fanning action of the flywheel blades cools you down. The original air-resistance bike was the Schwinn Airdyne, and in recent years many companies such as Raleigh, Excel, Pro Form, and DP have entered the market with such bikes in the $400 to $800 range.

Many of these bikes offer upper body conditioning for the arms along with the lower body workout. Dual-action stationary bicycles incorporate movable handlebars to provide an efficient, simultaneous upper body workout. Exercise bicycles such as the Schwinn Airdyne also permit the use of just one system—either handlebars or pedals—at a time. This gives the home exerciser a choice of four options for a balanced upper and lower body workout program: (a) legs and hips alone; (b) arms and shoulders alone; (c) combined leg and arm effort; and (d) arms and upper torso.

Finally, there is the electromagnetic/electronic bike, which basically consists of a steel flywheel surrounded by a series of magnets, all enclosed in the bike's housing. An electronic mechanism tells the magnets to apply more or less resistance to the flywheel. Because the resistance is controlled by a magnetic field, resistance changes are smooth. Many of these bikes offer control panels that show distance covered, calories burned, fitness scores, heart rate, and course profiles. Today's fitness enthusiasts like being able to program workouts because it makes exercising more fun and can be motivational, but don't be attracted by gimmicky electronics that don't add value to your workouts.

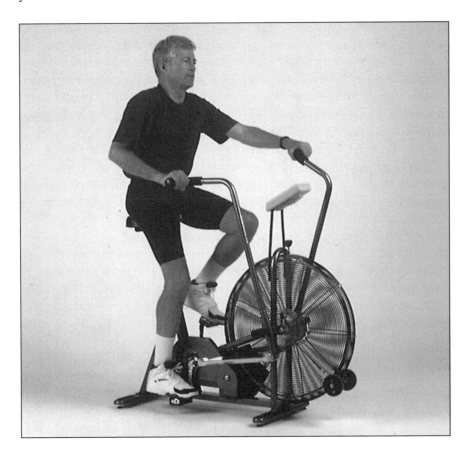

## A LAID-BACK WORKOUT

As you are reading this chapter, the next revolution in stationary bikes is taking place: the recumbent bike. These bikes, which place the exerciser in a reclined or semireclined position, come in both wind-resistance and electromagnetic-resistance models.

Harvey Newton, Director of Programs for the National Strength and Conditioning Association, states that recumbent bicycles are extremely comfortable to use and ideal for individuals wanting or needing a change from standard upright seating. A recumbent position also makes it possible to perform other activities while working out—such as reading or watching television. This makes it easier for the individual to integrate exercise into his or her lifestyle and realize personal fitness goals more quickly.

Exercising with a tired back in an uncomfortable position turns many people off to upright stationary bikes. Most individuals interested in purchasing a stationary bike are looking for comfort, security, and a quality workout. Finding a seat that is comfortable is probably the most difficult part of shopping for a stationary bike, so the recumbent, with its chairlike seat, is likely to win a lot of fans.

Recumbent bikes aren't prohibitively expensive, either. The Schwinn® Personal Trainer 205, for example, has a suggested retail price of about $349. Precor and other companies offer models for less than $450.

Don't dismiss the recumbent bike as a mere luxury. Sales of recumbent bikes are on the increase, and retailers attribute much of their popularity to consumers with back problems, the severely overweight, and those who have difficulty with balance.

The recumbent position and the large bucket seat distribute weight more evenly over the lower back and buttocks, making recumbent bikes an excellent choice for those with back problems. Lower body musculoskeletal fitness is critical to the maintenance of functional mobility in those with back pain, so orthopedically safe weight-bearing exercise is invaluable.

For severely overweight individuals, a semirecumbent position is more comfortable because the seat supports the entire pelvis and lumbar spine, preventing contact point fatigue during workouts. For those with orthopedic/musculoskeletal limitations, recumbents eliminate potentially troublesome hip and knee hyperextension by positioning the legs slightly below the waist. For many, they also eliminate the unnatural forward lean and upward pushing sensation on the arms and shoulders experienced on upright stationary bikes.

Physically handicapped individuals and seniors with balance problems will find the recumbent easier than trying to straddle an upright bike. Because the seat is the same height as a regular chair, recumbents are easier to get into and out of, making them safer and more inviting. Those who suffer from arthritis will also find the comfort of recumbent cycling more rewarding than exercise on an upright bike, treadmill, or rowing machine.

Recumbents are ideal for individuals with extremely low fitness levels because they require less energy cost at low workloads than upright cycling. They are also ideal for cardiac rehabilitation because, at equal work loads, patients need not work as hard to get the same benefit from a recumbent as from a stationary bike. The heart doesn't have to fight gravity to pump blood, so the user's heart rate and blood pressure are lower.

Finally, recumbents offer a change of pace for cyclists because they work slightly different muscle groups of the legs and work the buttock and hamstring muscles more than an upright bike. They also provide a winter training alternative for those individuals who commute or exercise on outdoor recumbent bikes as well as the added advantage of training specificity in the recumbent position.

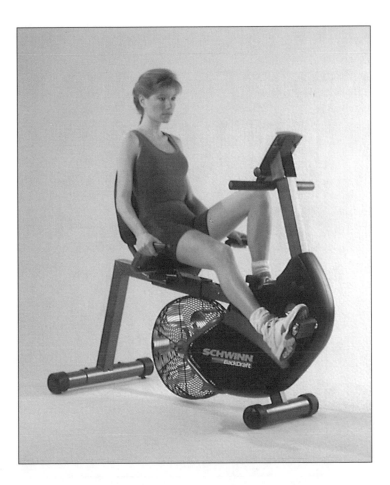

# WIND AND MAGNETIC TRAINERS

The invention of the wind trainer has brightened indoor training for thousands of fitness enthusiasts because they can now train on their regular road bike indoors. In fact, different size bikes can be installed easily, allowing family members to share the same machine.

Wind trainers have two fan units with slotted blades that churn the air. Magnetic trainers have powerful magnets and a nonconductive disk that produces resistance and dissipates energy as heat. Performance mag trainers have several resistance settings (low to high) and are controlled by a bar-mounted lever.

The wind trainer's greatest advantage for indoor training is that it closely mimics the exponential increases in wind resistance experienced on the road. For example, if you were to increase your speed on the wind-load simulator from 15 to 30 mph, you would need to increase your power output by a factor of about eight to reach

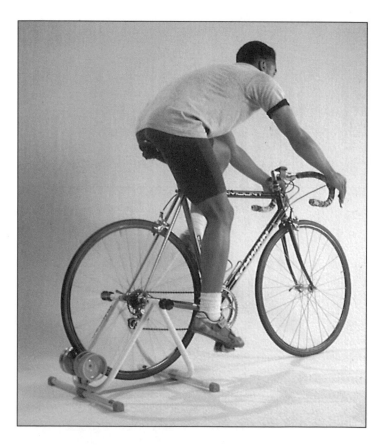

30 mph. The disadvantages of wind trainers are the noise generated by the fans and the lack of resistance adjustment.

With magnetic resistance units, resistance increases in direct proportion to speed, which is less realistic than with wind-load simulators; however, they do provide enough drag to elevate your heart rate. Variable-resistance magnetic units incorporate a small, precisely weighted flywheel that produces a slight coasting sensation and helps you pedal through the dead spots in your pedal stroke for a more realistic road feel. Advantages of magnetic trainers over the wind trainer include reduced noise levels and the ability to vary resistance.

## JOHNNY G. SPINNER™

You might have heard of "Spinning[R]" workouts, where people ride stationary bikes (usually to loud, energetic music) in a class led by an instructor, much like an aerobics class. The Johnny G. Spinner™ bike by Schwinn is designed to duplicate real riding as much as possible: Saddles and handlebars are adjustable; the fixed gear is attached to a flywheel, encouraging a smooth stroke; and resistance is easily adjusted to simulate hills and intervals. This program has benefits—it does not require rhythm or a good sense of balance, there are no inclement weather concerns or traffic obstacles, and all riders will arrive at the finish line at the same time.

You don't need an instructor to do your own workout, though. With your bike and a stereo, you can create workouts to fit your mood. Spinning[R] is a great, low-impact way to add excitement and variety to your home fitness routine.

# BICYCLE FIT

Most stationary bicycles come in one size that fits all. Once set up in your home gym, adjust it to fit you, not the other way around. Chronic injuries and much discomfort have been caused by improper positioning, especially by having the saddle too high or too low.

## SEAT HEIGHT

The saddle should be positioned high enough so that when the pedal is at the bottom of the stroke and the ball of your foot is on the pedal, your knee has a slight bend in it. Your hips should not move from side to side as you pedal, and you should never have to stretch your leg to reach the pedal at the bottom of the stroke.

Always wear the same shoes when riding your bike—a quarter of an inch can make a big difference in knee extension. If you add a pad to your saddle, lower it to compensate for the added thickness.

Many bicycles only allow about an inch change in saddle position by moving a pin from one hole to another. Move the saddle up or down slightly rather than risk injury by riding with the saddle too low or too high.

There is as much variation in bicycle saddles as there is in bicycle types—so no one seat is going to fit everyone. Generally speaking, women's seat bones are farther apart than men's, but some men have seat bones that are farther apart than women's. A study conducted by

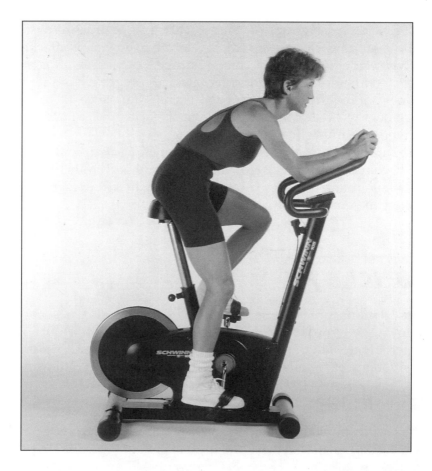

Dr. Martha Jack at Washington State University found a difference of 4 inches in the distance between seat bones in over 50 women tested. Thus, some would be comfortable on a men's narrow saddle and others would need the widest saddle available on the market.

Wide tractor-type saddles often have firm padding, which undoes the cushioning effect, and their width can often chafe the inner surface of the thighs. What feels comfortable for the first 10 minutes can hurt a lot after 30 minutes. Pressure and numbing that may be unnoticeable at first can become unbearable after 30 minutes. Adding a gel saddle pad to the seat will add height, which means you will have to readjust your seat height.

Sometimes pressure problems in the crotch area can be solved by changing the angle of the seat. Women seem to be comfortable with the saddle level or tilted slightly downward (too much tilting puts a lot of pressure on your hands) and men with it tilted slightly upward.

If you have made all the adjustments possible on your bike and are still uncomfortable, try purchasing a pair of high-quality padded cycling shorts or take the saddle and seat post to your bike shop and get a new seat that will fit the post. New foam-padded, anatomical saddles are available in men's and women's widths that have hollows positioned to correspond to human pressure points.

## FORE AND AFT POSITION OF THE SADDLE

With the balls of your feet on the pedal and the pedals in a horizontal position—at 3 o'clock and 9 o'clock—a plumb line dropped from just behind the kneecap on the outside of your forward knee should pass through the axle of the pedal.

Your knee should be over the axle of the pedal. If the seat is too far forward, your knee will bend more at the top of the pedal stroke and put a lot of pressure on the inside of your kneecap. If it is too far back, the hamstrings at the back of your leg will be stretched too much. Remember, by loosening the bolt under the saddle, the seat can be moved forward or backward on its rails.

When the saddle is lowered or raised, it also moves forward or backward. How much it moves depends on the angle of the seat tube, which depends on the design of your stationary bicycle.

If individuals with widely differing leg lengths and fore/aft positions are to use the bicycle, more than one seat post may have to be used to ensure proper saddle height and fore/aft positioning. In addition, the same saddle or saddle tilt may not be comfortable for all individuals.

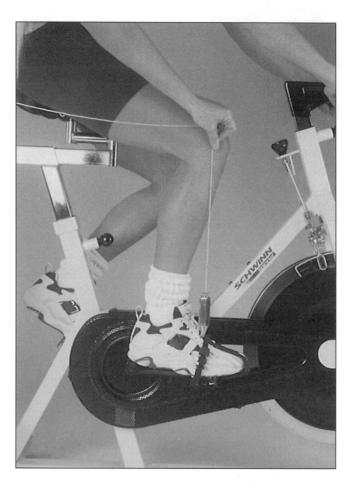

## HANDLEBAR POSITION

You should not have to stretch to reach the handlebars, nor should you be confined by having them too close to your body. Your elbows should be bent slightly, and you should be able to reach the handlebars from a comfortable upright position.

## PEDAL FIT

The ball of your foot, not the instep, should be on the pedal. If using toe clips and straps, make sure that they do not force your feet into an unnatural angle. Not everyone's feet point straight ahead, and if your try to force them to, you may put undue stress on your knees.

Wear either bicycle touring shoes or walking shoes with a firm bottom. Do not wear shoes with too much cushioning.

# INDOOR WORKOUTS

As with all exercise, remember to spend a few minutes warming up and cooling down after each session on the bicycle. Cycling indoors is much different from cycling outdoors because you don't have the wind to keep you cool. Within 5 minutes, you'll be overheated if you don't have a cooling system, so I recommend using a fan. You might also consider riding in the coolest part of the house. Many cyclists set up their stationary bikes in an unheated part of their home such as a garage or basement. Also, remember to fill your water bottle before starting your workout.

To make your workouts more enjoyable, be creative. Make a couple of training tapes of your favorite songs (preferably something with a strong beat), and put on your headphones when you start to pedal. Use a bike computer to monitor your progress, keeping a log of times, distances, and speeds, or use a heart rate monitor to track your workout level. By keeping your training fun, you can avoid burnout and improve your cycling skills.

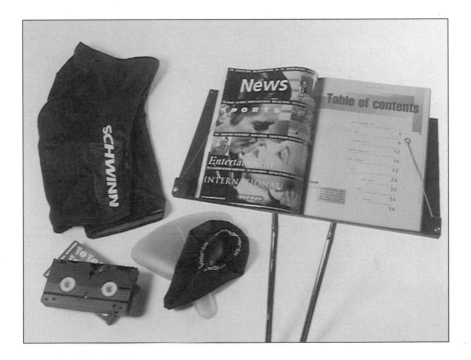

Many people position their exercise bikes in front of a TV so they can watch their favorite show or video while riding. Several companies have produced excellent videos and audiotapes just for use while exercising on a stationary bike. A company called Videocycle offers a series of tapes of scenic places that allow the rider to enjoy the sense of riding in the countryside. One of the leaders in the audio market is Medical & Sports Music Institute of America, whose audiotapes allow individuals to pace their workouts at their desired rhythm and target heart rate.

For general conditioning, find a resistance that elevates your heart rate into your training zone. After your warm-up, increase your speed to 80 to 95 rpm with your heart rate at no more than 85 percent of your maximum.

Don't be intimidated by terms such as kilopound meters (kpm), kilopounds (kp), or watts (W). Depending on the manufacturer,

### Table 7.1   Workload/Energy Equivalents

| Work Performance | | | Energy Equivalents | | Walk/Run Equivalents | |
|---|---|---|---|---|---|---|
| Watts | kp | kpm/min | Calories Min | Hr | Min/mile | mph |
| 25 | 0.5 | 150 | 3.0 | 180 | 30 | 2 |
| 50 | 1.0 | 300 | 4.5 | 270 | 20 | 3 |
| 75 | 1.5 | 450 | 6.0 | 360 | | |
| 100 | 2.0 | 600 | 7.5 | 450 | 13 | 4.5 |
| 125 | 2.5 | 750 | 9.0 | 540 | | |
| 150 | 3.0 | 900 | 10.5 | 630 | 10 | 6 |
| 175 | 3.5 | 1050 | 12.0 | 720 | | |
| 200 | 4.0 | 1200 | 14.0 | 840 | 8 | 7.5 |
| 225 | 4.5 | 1350 | 15.0 | 900 | | |
| 250 | 5.0 | 1500 | 17.0 | 1020 | 7 | 8.5 |
| 275 | 5.5 | 1650 | 18.0 | 1080 | | |
| 300 | 6.0 | 1800 | 20.0 | 1200 | 6 | 10.0 |

workload settings are expressed in watts, calories, kilopound meters, or horsepower. The key is to set the resistance (workload) at a level that will stress your heart and lungs sufficiently to increase your fitness. It is important to adjust the load to ensure a training stimulus in the 60 to 85 percent target heart rate range. Use the programs outlined by the machine you are using or the accompanying workload equivalent table (see Table 7.1) to help you design a personalized training program and to obtain information on the load setting you are using.

A final tip: Ride your trainer only every other day; otherwise, you are likely to get stale. On days when you don't ride, get your aerobic workout by skiing or stepping. You can ski or lift weights the same day you ride.

The following are examples of several workouts that can be used on stationary bicycles. Variations of these workouts can also be used on stair climbers and treadmills.

## PYRAMID WORKOUT

Start with 10 minutes of hard effort followed by 2 minutes of easy spinning for recovery. The next interval should be 8 minutes hard, 2 minutes easy. Each hard interval should decrease by 2 minutes but increase slightly in intensity. The easy 2-minute intervals should remain the same. End the workout when you reach intervals of 2 minutes hard and 2 minutes easy.

## HILL WORKOUT

Ride using progressively higher resistances. Start with a relatively low resistance and ride for 1 to 2 minutes, then shift to the next higher resistance, and so on (keeping the same cadence throughout exercise). After you have finished riding at the highest resistance you plan to ride, reverse the process by riding back down the hill (at progressively lower resistances). Usually, riding four to five workloads is sufficient for a good workout.

There are dozens of variations of the above workout. High resistance, low resistance, back to high, up two workloads, down one, and so on. You can also vary the cadence, increasing it to 110 to 120 rpm for a minute or so but always keeping it above 80 rpm.

## HEART RATE ZONE WORKOUT

Here's a good aerobic workout if you want to do an endurance ride in a specific heart rate zone (for example, between 75 and 80 percent of MHR).

Warm up for about 5 minutes, starting with low to moderate resistance, and gradually increase your speed or workload until your heart rate is at 75 percent of your maximum. For the next 30 minutes, keep your heart rate within 75 to 80 percent of the target range you calculated before getting on the bike. The challenge of this workout is to keep your heart rate in the target zone. If it falls below or rises above this zone, increase or decrease your effort.

Cool down for 5 to 10 minutes until your heart rate has dropped to below 60 percent of maximum.

## LADDER WORKOUT

The 10 minute ascending-descending ladder bicycle workout can be used on busy days or in the middle of a weight workout. Start with a 5-minute warm-up at low resistance. At the end of your warm-up, your heart rate should be at 60 percent of MHR. Over the next 10 minutes, slowly increase the resistance as you attempt to attain the desired training heart rate at each minute.

Minute 1 at 65 percent of MHR

Minute 2 at 70 percent of MHR

Minute 3 at 75 percent of MHR

Minute 4 at 80 percent of MHR

Minute 5 at 85 percent of MHR

Minute 6 at 85 percent of MHR

Minute 7 at 80 percent of MHR

Minute 8 at 75 percent of MHR

Minute 9 at 70 percent of MHR

Minute 10 at 65 percent of MHR

Five minute cool-down, low resistance

This program is not cut in stone; don't be afraid to modify the intensity levels as needed.

## ✓ INJURY PREVENTION

Don't hyperextend your leg when pedaling on the downstroke. Adjust the seat so you can maintain a slight bend in your knee.

Keep your small children away from moving parts, so fingers do not become caught in fan blades, rubber bands, or spinning wheels.

Don't dismount the stationary bicycle until the pedals and arms (if using a dual-action bicycle) have come to a complete stop.

# THE FINAL SPIN

A stationary bicycle is a wonderful adjunct to an exercise program. With it you can develop a stronger heart, strengthen leg muscles, and burn calories. In addition, using a stationary bike does not require bearing your total body weight on your feet, ankles, knees, or hips and can enable you to exercise even if you have chronic medical problems in these areas.

A final word about stationary bikes. You may encounter some flak from your friends who insist that road riding is the only way to cycle. But take heart. As pointed out in this chapter, you can use your stationary bike not only to keep in shape but to supplement your road riding all year round.

Besides, it's even trendy. A local airline magazine recently advertised the opening of a plush new hotel in New York with the latest luxuries. When asked what the innovation was (An in-room sauna? A fax in every room?), the management replied somewhat stuffily: "Of course not. We've supplied each room with something even better . . . exercise bikes!"

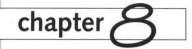

# chapter 8

# Stair Climbing

## Julie A. Spotts, BSEM

*A*s the 1980s got under way, so did a new craze in fitness. In health clubs across the country, lines were forming in front of the newest piece of exercise equipment: the stair-climbing machine. The stair climber quickly grew in popularity, and more than 10 years later it is still a favorite piece of aerobic equipment.

Stair climbing is not a new idea, however. For years, coaches everywhere used bleacher stands and stairs to condition their athletes. Although there was no research to back up the efficacy of these training techniques, coaches knew that stair climbing produced positive results. Today research shows that a fitness program using stair-climbing machines can produce significant aerobic benefits and is a safer alternative than climbing bleachers or stairwells.

Stair climbing's primary purpose is to provide aerobic conditioning: strengthening the heart and burning calories to reduce fat. It also tones your calves, thighs, and buttocks. But exercise bikes and treadmills can offer the same benefits, so why buy a stair climber? There are several reasons. First, stair climbing requires a higher metabolic equivalent (MET), or power requirement, than cycling or running. (A MET correlates the amount of energy required to perform a specific activity with that needed in a resting state.) In simple terms, stair climbing consumes more calories per workout than an equal amount of time spent on a treadmill or exercise bike.

Second, it is a lower impact alternative to running. Finally, stair climbing offers a refreshing change from the saddle sores associated with riding an exercise bike.

# CHOOSING THE RIGHT STAIR CLIMBER FOR YOU

Once you have decided to purchase a stair climber, the choices may seem overwhelming. To help narrow your options, first identify the features that are most important to you. The answers to the following questions will help determine the type or class of machine you will need.

1. How much money do you have to spend?
2. How much floor space is available for the machine?
3. Do you want a computer that accurately calculates calories burned, power output, and/or heart rate?
4. Do you want a computer to control and vary the resistance of the machine?
5. Do you want independent or dependent stepping action?

Usually, price will be the biggest factor in your decision. No need to worry, though, as there are some very reasonably priced, high-quality stair climbers on the market today.

One way to distinguish between stair climbers is according to whether the mechanical action of the stepping pedals is dependent or independent. In a stair climber with dependent action, the right and left pedals are tied together such that when the user pushes down the right pedal, the left pedal comes up, and vice versa. The most popular line of dependent-action stair climbers in health clubs today is manufactured by Life Fitness. Both Precor and Tunturi manufacture dependent-action stair climbers that are designed for home use. These machines make it easier to develop a rhythm, which can be beneficial for beginners.

Stair climbers with pedals that move independently eliminate the user's ability to shift his or her weight from side to side to keep the pedals moving (an action that is possible on stair climbers with dependent action). This side-to-side shifting can reduce the effectiveness of a workout. Thus, stair climbers with independent pedal action can minimize the user's ability to cheat his or her workout. More importantly, research has shown that independent-action stair climbers reduce the risk of orthopedic trauma compared to stepping on dependent-action stair climbers or climbing stairwells. Schwinn Cycling & Fitness, Inc. has developed a line of independent-action stair climbing machines designed for home and health club use.

# CLASSES OF STAIR CLIMBERS

For simplicity, stair-climbing machines can be classified into three different categories: cylinder-driven, wind-driven, and computer-controlled. In general, you can find both independent- and dependent-action stair climbers in all three categories.

## CYLINDER-DRIVEN STAIR CLIMBERS

The most common type of stair climbers in the lower price market are those with cylinders that use air or hydraulic fluid to provide resistance. Some machines allow you to change the resistance setting on the cylinder. This type of machine is highly recommended because, as your stepping ability increases, so will your need for various resistance settings.

If you are looking for independent stepping action, you will probably have to pay slightly more for your machine. With independent-action stair climbers, the pedals are not tied together with a belt or cable, so the cylinders are required to bear the full load of the user. Thus, you will want to buy a stair climber with heavy-duty cylinders. A rule of thumb is the thicker or greater the outer diameter of the cylinder, the greater the load capacity. Schwinn Cycling and Fitness carries an independent-action cylinder-driven stair climber for approximately $299. Retail prices run between $250 and $600 for an independent-action cylinder-driven stair climber and between $180 and $300 for a dependent-action cylinder-driven stair climber.

Because the resistance of these machines is not controlled by a computer, most units come with simple programs that keep track of your workout time, total number of steps, and approximate distance climbed. Some will also calculate the average number of calories burned for the number of steps you have climbed.

One last note about cylinder-driven stair climbers. The market is now supplying some dual-action stair climbers that also train the upper body. Although these machines offer an improved total body workout, you will notice the difference in the sticker price. An inexpensive alternative is to buy a set of hand weights and develop your own upper body workout.

## WIND-DRIVEN STAIR CLIMBERS

The next major category of stair climbers are those that use a fan to provide resistance. The user varies the resistance by speeding up or slowing down the stepping rate (i.e., the slower the step rate, the lower the resistance). These machines cost more than cylinder-driven stair climbers but are more durable. The cooling effect of the fan is an added benefit. Ultra Fit manufactures a wind-driven stair climber that retails for approximately $650. This unit combines a fan with a friction belt for even more variability in resistance.

## COMPUTER-CONTROLLED STAIR CLIMBERS

These stair climbers use computers to control the resistance provided by a brake. One advantage of this type of system is that resistance changes can occur without input from the user. With this feature, preprogrammed workouts can be selected at the beginning of a session. The computer can simulate changes in speed or force as the user encounters hills or valleys. These types of programs add variety to your workout and help alleviate boredom. Another advantage of computer-controlled stair climbers is that they provide more accurate feedback on calorie consumption and energy expenditure.

Computer-controlled machines are available with various features and in many price categories, but an important differentiator is the type of braking mechanism used. Your choice of brake will depend on which features you require. Table 8.1 provides general guidelines for brake selection.

The 4000 PT, manufactured by Stair Master, is an example of an alternator-driven computer-controlled stair climber. This model retails for approximately $2,195. A more economical model manufactured by Schwinn Cycling and Fitness retails for approximately $1,299. This model, the CI-330, is driven with an electromagnetic brake.

### Table 8.1   Brake Selection for Computer-Controlled Stair Climbers

| Braking Mechanism | Advantages | Disadvantages |
| --- | --- | --- |
| Eddy current | Economical | Shorter warranty life |
| Electromagnetic | Durable<br>Fairly accurate power output readings | May not provide enough resistance for a user over 250 lb |
| Alternator | Very durable | Power readings are inaccurate unless machine is calibrated |

Although the three categories just discussed cover the majority of stair climbers now available, there is one other type of machine that should be mentioned. A few brands of stair climbers are designed to mimic escalator stairs. The effect of these machines is similar to actually climbing stairs, but they are more difficult to use because they require better rhythm. On these machines, slips can easily turn into injuries. Furthermore, these machines are typically designed for institutional use and thus are fairly expensive. Table 8.2 summarizes the major categories of stair-climbing machines.

### Table 8.2   Stair Climbers and Their Features

| Type of Stair Climber | Price | Floor Space | Accurate Readouts | Predicted Life |
| --- | --- | --- | --- | --- |
| Cylinder-driven | Most economical ($200-$600) | Minimal | Time and step rate accurate<br>All other readouts are approximate | Not very durable |
| Wind-driven | Moderately priced ($500-$700) | Moderate | Moderately accurate | Moderately durable |
| Computer-controlled | Expensive ($800-$3500) | Normally require most floor space | Typically accurate readings | Very durable depending on braking mechanism |

# CORRECT STEPPING PROCEDURE

Although stair climbers have become very popular, few people know about or use the correct posture or stance to maximize their workouts and minimize injuries. Taking time to learn how to use your stair climber properly from the start will help you avoid injury and increase the effectiveness of your workout.

The most common mistake in stair climbing is using your arms to support your body weight. This method decreases the amount of weight you are lifting with each step, thus decreasing the amount of energy you expend during the workout. Research has shown that you can increase your oxygen consumption rate by up to 25 percent by eliminating arm support. An arm-weighted position can also cause unnecessary wrist and elbow strain. To avoid this problem and

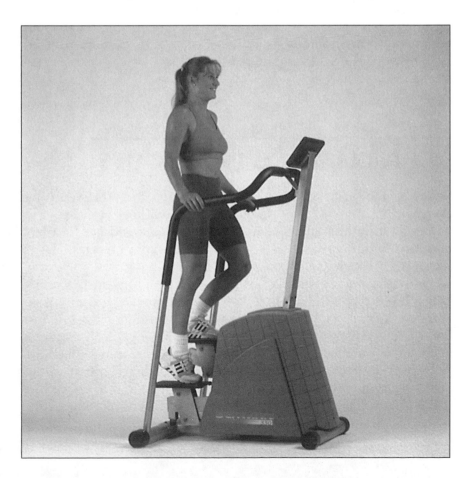

increase your productivity, use the handlebars for stability only. In fact, once you have mastered the stepping motion, stop using the handlebar and add hand weights to your stepping regime. This will exercise your upper body and increase your caloric consumption.

The second most common mistake is to lean over the handlebars while stepping. Again, you are unweighting your lower body and decreasing the effectiveness of your workout. This position can also strain your lower back. To avoid this problem, stand up straight with your upper body in the same vertical plane as your hips and legs.

Another type of injury that can result from stair climbing usually occurs during the bottom of the pedal stroke, when the knee is fully extended. If the machine is not designed properly, the knee can go beyond full extension into slight hyperextension, resulting in injury. When purchasing a stair climber, verify that the machine is designed to allow proper positioning of the knee.

A further note on hyperextension injuries and equipment design: More expensive models incorporate self-leveling pedals that remain horizontal throughout the entire range of motion. If you can afford such models, the self-leveling pedals will reduce the risk of knee injury.

# STAIR-CLIMBING WORKOUTS

Before beginning any exercise program, always start with stretching exercises. Chapter 4 gives suggestions on various stretches and warm-up routines. After adequate stretching, spend the first few minutes of your workout slowly warming up your muscles. This is one of the most effective ways to prevent strain injuries.

The most important aspect of any exercise program is variety, which helps increase both your workout frequency and duration. Watching television, listening to music, or reading a magazine can help distract you and make the workout more enjoyable. For variety, add cycling, running, or weight training to your workout schedule.

To spice up your stair climbing workout, change your stepping positions frequently. Wide foot pedals allow you to move your feet to different positions to exercise different muscle groups. Begin your

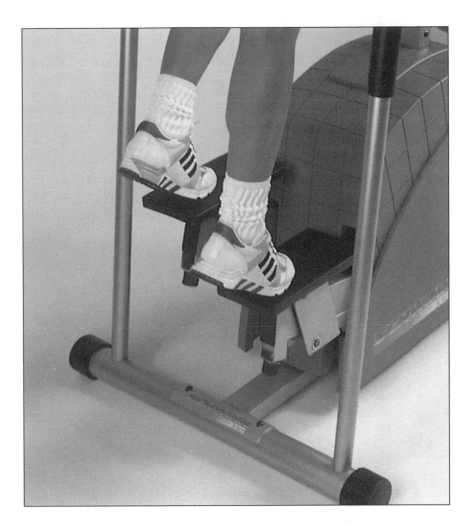

workout in a flat-footed position with your feet pointing forward. Next, move your feet to the edges of the pedals and stand on the ball of each foot. As you become more comfortable with your stair climber, you can even ride the machine backward.

Whichever position you choose for your workout, the main objective of stair climbing (as with any type of aerobic training) is to elevate your heart rate to within 60 to 85 percent of your maximum. The exact choice will depend on the training effect you desire. See chapter 3 for recommended heart rate training zones.

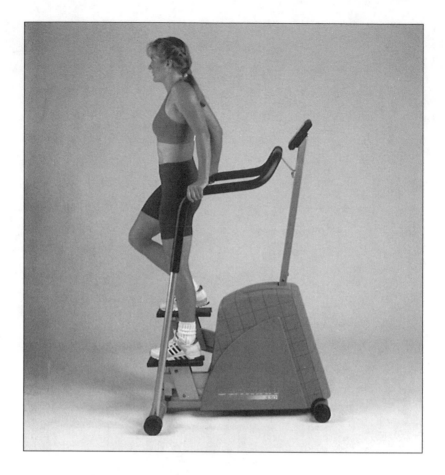

The more sophisticated stair climbers provide a readout of watts or horsepower, or the amount of energy the user is expending to maintain the motion over time. This readout is used mostly in hospitals and rehabilitation centers. Not all computers have accurate readings, so shop carefully if you require a machine with this feature.

Some of the more expensive computer-controlled stair climbers are equipped with workout programs for your selection. If one of these machines is not in your price range, try using a clock and your heart rate or step rate to make up your own workout programs. The following are some sample workouts.

## THE 30 MINUTE WORKOUT

The goal of this workout is to vary your step rate to keep within a target heart rate zone (i.e., the higher the step rate, the higher the heart rate). Refer to chapter 3 on how to determine your maximum heart rate. The chart below shows the percentage of MHR to be maintained for each cumulative time specified throughout the workout. (For example, at 14 minutes into your workout you will maintain a heart rate that is 70% of your maximum.)

| Program time (minutes) | Target heart rate |
| --- | --- |
| 0:00 to 10:00 | 60 percent of MHR |
| 10:01 to 12:00 | 70 percent of MHR |
| 12:01 to 13:00 | Return to original step rate |
| 13:01 to 15:00 | 70 percent of MHR |
| 15:01 to 16:00 | Return to original step rate |
| 16:01 to 18:00 | 75 percent of MHR |
| 18:01 to 19:00 | Return to original step rate |
| 19:01 to 21:00 | 75 percent of MHR |
| 21:01 to 22:00 | Return to original step rate |
| 22:01 to 24:00 | 80 percent of MHR |
| 24:01 to 25:00 | Return to original step rate |
| 25:01 to 27:00 | 80 percent of MHR |
| 27:01 to 30:00 | Return to original step rate |

## UPPER BODY WORKOUT

For this workout, you will need hand weights (a plastic container filled with water or sand works just as well). Begin your workout by warming up using leg action only. Next, add upper body exercises for 1 minute, followed by 1 minute of leg action only. Continue alternating this sequence until the end of your workout. Don't forget to cool down by stepping only. The upper body exercises can consist of biceps curls, with palms up or down, or synchronized arm swings (similar to your arm motion during walking).

## CONSTANT-RESISTANCE WORKOUT

Begin your program with a 5-minute warm-up period. Then, starting with a low step rate, gradually work up to a step rate that brings your heart rate to 75 percent of your MHR. Move your feet to the back of the pedals and begin stepping on the balls of each foot. Without changing the resistance setting on the machine, begin taking shallow, quick steps for 3 minutes. Follow this by returning to the original flat-footed position in the middle of the pedal and take deep, slow steps for 1 minute. Repeat intervals of 3 minutes of shallow, quick steps followed by 1 minute of deep, slow steps for the duration of your program time. Follow your program with a cool-down that returns your heart rate to 60 percent of your MHR.

## ✓ INJURY PREVENTION

Always stretch before working out.

Warm up and cool down for the first and last few minutes of your workout.

Stand straight when stepping.

Do not lean forward over the handlebars or support your weight with them.

Avoid hyperextension of the knee at the bottom of the pedal stroke.

Keep children and pets away from the machine while in use. Fingers can get caught in the fan blades of wind-driven mechanisms as well as beneath the pedal arms when in motion.

# THE FINAL STEP

If you still think you can fulfill your stepping needs by running the bleachers or climbing the back stairwell at work, consider the advantages of a stair-climbing machine. You will greatly reduce the risk of missing a step and slamming your face into the bleachers. More importantly, you will be able to track and monitor your workouts more effectively, reduce your chances of injury, and enjoy significant cardiovascular conditioning while making the exercise much more convenient and enjoyable.

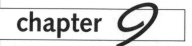

# Trekking on Treadmills

**Edmund R. Burke, PhD**

With prices ranging from $150 for nonmotorized models to $4,000 for motorized models, and features that can simulate everything from walking trails to mountain runs, the array of treadmill choices available to the home exerciser is overwhelming. Many have taken a second look at treadmills and found they may be the most versatile aerobic exercise machine around.

There are two basic kinds of treadmills: manual and electric. On a manual treadmill, you provide the power. As you walk or run, your feet push the tread surface back over a smooth surface or a series of rollers. The treadmill speeds up and slows down according to your effort. With a motorized treadmill, on the other hand, you select the speed you want and a motor drives the belt at that speed. Then it's your challenge to walk or run fast enough to stay in one place.

On most treadmills, both manual and electric, the elevation angle can be adjusted to simulate uphill exercise. If you've never learned to appreciate the difference a few degrees of slope can make, it will only take one session on an elevated treadmill to make a believer out of you.

Improved tread surface is just one of the reasons many exercisers are taking to treadmills. With their cushioned decks, treadmills absorb up to 40 percent of the impact of running on roads. Choosing a treadmill is like buying a new car—it depends as much on the driver as on the machine itself. A treadmill that feels soft to someone who runs on the balls of their feet may be perfect for a heavy heel-to-toe runner. Try at least three different models before buying; walk or run on each for a couple of minutes to find the unit that best suits your walking or running style.

# MOTORIZED TREADMILLS

Few high-quality motorized treadmills retail for under $1,000. You can buy one for less, but it's not likely to perform the way you would like. Most inexpensive treadmills are better suited for walking than for running. Schwinn Cycling and Fitness currently produces one home model, the Home Trainer 615 treadmill, for about $1,900 with a continuous 1.5-horsepower motor and a cushioned deck. The Life Fitness 3500 sells for approximately $2,350 and tops out at 9 mph. Buying a high-quality motorized treadmill—an absolute must for the serious fitness enthusiast—will generally cost you $1,000 or more; those that cost less are all too often noisy, poorly designed, uncomfortable, and can be unsafe to use. The payoff is that a good treadmill will provide you with many years of great aerobic exercise, making it one of the best home fitness investments.

Several factors separate the high-quality treadmills from the pretenders. Check the amount of power delivered. If you are running more than walking, look for a motor with at least a 1.5-horsepower continuous duty rating. To make sure a treadmill has enough power, set it to 2 mph and step on the belt; if it slows considerably under your weight, you're dealing with inferior machinery. Most home units use DC motors, whereas commercial treadmills may have either AC or DC. AC motors tend to be noisier and to draw more current; the latter means that an AC treadmill will likely require a dedicated power line.

Observe the continuous horsepower rating, which is the continuous power that a treadmill motor can reach and maintain under any load or no-load condition. This rating, which is the most powerful rating listed, is important to ensure concise, steady-state running.

Some manufacturers report only treadmill horsepower rating or peak horsepower rating. Be sure to compare apples to apples. Treadmill horsepower rating is the amount of horsepower a motor can reach under intermittent load conditions (approximately 70 to 80 percent of continuous horsepower rating). Peak horsepower rating is the absolute maximum horsepower a treadmill motor can reach under peak load conditions (approximately 50 to 60 percent of continuous horsepower rating).

Many treadmills feature panic buttons that bring the treadmill to a rapid halt. In combination with side or front rails, these stop buttons are designed to make the user feel more at ease while exercising.

A welded frame and deck construction is by far the most durable. Bolts and rivets will eventually rattle loose. Look for laminated decks that can be maintained simply by wiping away dust and debris from under the belt or with an occasional spray of silicone. Avoid machines that require regular waxing.

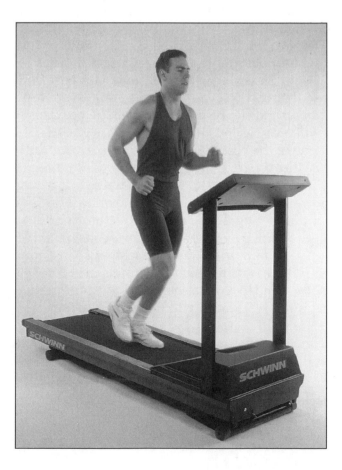

The standard walking or running surface is 18 inches wide by 51 to 54 inches long, which is sufficient for runners or walkers of normal height and average running proficiency. Extra-wide (20 inches or more) or extra-long (more than 54 inches) decks are recommended for those with extremely long strides or those who have disabilities. Two-ply belts are stronger and less likely to curl at the sides than one-ply belts.

Treadmills for walking range in speed from 0 or 0.5 mph up to around 5 or 6 mph, whereas those for jogging or running generally range from 0, 0.5, or 1 mph up to 8-12 mph. Operating a treadmill near maximum speed during every workout is a sure way to shorten motor life. Percentage of incline can range from a low of 0 to 2 percent to a high of 15 percent.

Electronic feedback displays of speed, time, and distance are generally standard on most treadmills. Some also display the number of calories burned and/or heart rate. In addition, most treadmills offer preset programs and the ability to save up to 10 personal programs, and some even record your workout history.

## Going Faster on the Beltway

If you do choose to walk or run fast on a treadmill, you might be deceived (but pleasantly so) by the results. Several studies have shown that it takes less energy to exercise at a given speed on an indoor treadmill than to exercise at the same speed outdoors. Why? Because there's less air resistance for you to cut through indoors.

You can make up for that loss by raising the elevation until you're working at the same heart rate as outdoors. If you normally exercise on flat roads, you'll need to set the treadmill at a 2 to 4 percent grade. If you walk or run on hilly terrain, you'll have to experiment, most likely using heart rate as a guide.

Most individuals find some solace in exercising indoors in the absence of distractions. With no variances in environment, it is easier to set a steady pace and concentrate on technique. Because a treadmill forces you to exercise at a steady pace, you'll be programmed for walking at a particular speed and what it should feel like when you return to the road again.

# MANUAL TREADMILLS

In the past, the price of a treadmill has been prohibitive for most home exercisers. But not anymore. A whole new breed of treadmills has arrived on the fitness market.

The new kids on the block are nonmotorized versions that cost between $150 and $600. What's different about these nonmotorized treadmills? New technology has given them a smoother ride. The new models are designed with heavy freewheels that help regulate the momentum of your foot power, creating a smoother, more flowing gait. If you are considering an inexpensive motorized treadmill, put that thought aside and buy a manual one instead, simply because they're less likely to break down.

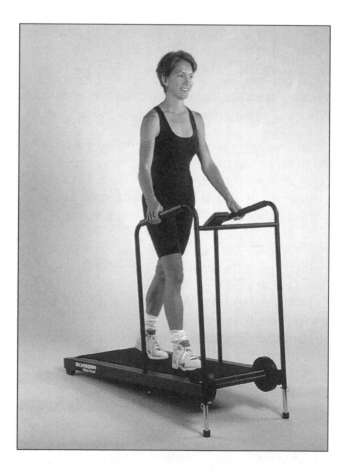

But make no mistake about it, these treadmills require hard work. They're all set at a slight incline to assist the treadmill action, so you're always walking slightly uphill. Manual treadmills have the disadvantage of being slower and more difficult to operate because the user powers the belt; if the exerciser begins to tire and slows down, the belt slows down too. On an electric model, the belt continues at the same speed, forcing the exerciser to keep going at that speed. With a nonmotorized treadmill, you have to challenge the machine; the motorized version challenges you. The choice will depend on what you are more comfortable with.

Two well-known manual treadmills in this category are the NordicTrack WalkFit for around $600 and the Easy Strider by Ultrafit for about $360. The WalkFit has poles that can be used to add an upper body workout. The Schwinn® Easy Tread treadmill has balanced, dual flywheels that provide plenty of inertia for a smooth, even response from this nonmotorized, self-propelled unit. These treadmills are ideal for anyone who is looking to get a great workout, day in and day out, without any mechanical problems.

# TREADMILL WORKOUTS

No one can dispute the popularity of treadmills as an indoor workout option. If you've never exercised on one, rest assured that you won't fly off the back of the moving belt. Most machines increase speed slowly, allowing you to progress from walking to jogging to running without undue stress. About the only difference you'll notice in walking or running on a treadmill versus outdoors is that when you get off and try to walk, you'll have sea legs. That sensation will go away after a few days. If you're unsteady, use the handrail and slow the speed until you feel comfortable dismounting.

To set everyone straight, here are a few basic tips even experienced exercisers should follow:

- Don't grip or lean on the handrails.
- Keep your arms moving while you exercise.
- Maintain good posture at all times.
- During warm weather, place a fan near the treadmill to keep you cool.

- Have a water bottle handy.
- If you plan to exercise for more than 20 minutes, crank up the music or tune the television to your favorite show.

You'll need to know your steady-state training speed to perform the following treadmill workouts. Start by setting the treadmill at its slowest speed and lowest elevation. Begin walking and increase your pace by 0.5 mph every 3 minutes until you feel warm, start breathing heavily, or feel as if you're pushing to maintain the pace. Reduce your speed by 0.5 mph and note the setting—that's your steady-state training pace. After at least 3 minutes at that pace, check your heart rate. It should be within 60 to 85 percent of your predicted maximum heart rate. If it's higher, reduce the speed.

## FLATS, INTERVALS, AND HILLS

Use this workout if you want to become a stronger, faster walker or runner. It will help you develop a better sense of pace and learn to deal with hills more efficiently. Best of all, it may help you set some new personal records when you return to the road.

**Warm-up:** 5 to 10 minutes at an easy pace; heart rate at 55 to 65 percent of maximum.

**Steady-State Segment:** 20 to 30 minutes; heart rate in the 65 to 85 percent range.

**Intervals:** Throw in several surges measured by distance, such as 1/8 to 3/4 mile, or time (30 seconds to 5 minutes, for a total of 20 to 30 minutes).

**Cool-down:** 5 to 10 minutes of easy jogging or walking, or until heart rate falls below 55 percent of maximum.

**Variation:** If you want to run hills, crank up the speed to your best 5- or 10-kilometer pace and slowly increase the incline. Use this variation as part of the interval segment.

## PYRAMID

This program divides your workout into several segments of equal length. The overall goal is to keep within your heart rate range, but by varying the grade and speed you will find it challenging. Your heart rate should be within 60 to 85 percent of your predicted or true MHR. You should begin the exercise session after warming up at your steady-state speed (discussed previously).

**Warm-up:** Walk or jog slowly for 5 to 10 minutes.

3 to 4 minutes: Flat grade at steady-state speed.

3 to 4 minutes: Increase grade to 2 percent; decrease speed by 0.5 mph.

3 to 4 minutes: Increase grade to 4 percent; decrease speed by 0.5 mph.

3 to 4 minutes: Increase grade to 6 percent; decrease speed by 0.5 mph.

3 to 4 minutes: Decrease grade to 4 percent; increase speed by 0.5 mph.

3 to 4 minutes: Decrease grade to 2 percent; increase speed by 0.5 mph.

**Cool-down:** Gradually return to a slow walk after 5 to 10 minutes.

## STRENGTH CIRCUIT

If you own resistance training equipment, consider alternating a 10-minute stint on the treadmill with a 10- to 15-minute strength training circuit. On a weight machine or free weights, do four to five different exercises, one to two sets each of 10 repetitions; return to the treadmill after each exercise, walking or running for several minutes between sets so that your heart rate remains somewhat elevated. Also, focus each successive exercise on a different body part, preferably one as far as possible from the previous body part exercised. This increases the workout for your heart. This same workout can be used if exercising on a stationary bike, skier, or stair climber, or if you have more than one, rotate between aerobic machines.

## ACCELERATE AND DECELERATE

Intervals of hard work train you to exercise at a higher intensity, and the rest periods lessen your risk of injury. To make this workout harder, shorten the recovery period by 30 seconds.

**Warm-up:** Walk or jog slowly for 5 to 10 minutes.

3 to 4 minutes: Increase the speed to 0.25 or 0.5 mph above your steady-state speed.

3 to 4 minutes: Decrease speed to a slow walk or jog (recovery speed).

3 to 4 minutes: Increase speed to steady-state speed on a 2 percent grade.

3 to 4 minutes: Decrease speed by at least 0.5 mph, but maintain grade.

3 to 4 minutes: Increase speed to 0.25 or 0.5 mph above steady-state speed.

3 to 4 minutes: Return to recovery speed.

3 to 4 minutes: Increase speed to steady-state speed on a 2 percent grade.

3 to 4 minutes: Return to recovery speed.

**Cool-down:** Gradually return to a walk after 5 to 10 minutes.

## THE 10-4 WORKOUT

This workout gets its name from its 10-4 pattern, a familiar phrase to those of you who use a two-way radio.

**Warm-up:** Walk or jog slowly for 10 minutes.

10 minutes: Walk or run at a predetermined heart rate or preselected pace; gradually increase the speed until you reach your predetermined heart rate.

4 minutes: Walk or jog to recover.

10 minutes: Surge again at your predetermined heart rate or selected pace.

4 minutes: Walk or jog to recover.

**Cool-down:** Complete the workout with 10 minutes of easy cool-down walking or running.

## ✓ INJURY PREVENTION

Make sure you wear the safety shutoff strap that connects to your shirt or shorts if your treadmill comes equipped with one. This automatically shuts off the machine if you happen to slip or fall.

Use the handrails for extra security when mounting, working out, or dismounting.

If you have bad knees or hips, consider purchasing a treadmill with built-in suspension for a shock-absorbing, low-impact workout.

Do not grip the handrails while exercising; learn to keep your arms moving while exercising.

# ROADLESS TRIP

Some fitness enthusiasts find treadmill running boring and tedious, complaining that there's nothing to look at but the four walls. Perhaps. But of the many benefits of treadmill walking and running, predictability may be its greatest virtue. The safety and security of walking or running in a well-lighted exercise room, the comfortable indoor temperature during winter months, and the reliable speed of the belt are just some of the pluses of indoor treadmill exercise.

Predictable does not have to mean boring. With a little imagination you can design a fitness program that is more precise and variable than your normal outdoor route. Also, with a nonmotorized or motorized treadmill you can control the pace to specifically target improving your walking or running pace or technique. For walkers and runners who balk at the sight of a stationary bike or ski machine, it's the best indoor exercise option.

Enter the treadmill, arguably the safest and most comfortable way to walk, jog, or run—either indoors or out.

# chapter 10

# Cross-Country Skiing Indoors

### Edmund R. Burke, PhD

*C*ross-country skiing is a nearly perfect form of exercise. By skiing and poling through the snow, you exercise your legs, arms, and upper body simultaneously, building muscular strength and increasing aerobic fitness. Cross-country ski machines seek to emulate cross-country skiing by imitating the sport's distinctive diagonal striding: The left arm moves forward as the left leg moves back, and vice versa.

The typical machine has two sliding boards or footpads for skis. The "poles" are either a pair of handles attached to a rope-and-pulley system or a full-length lever arm, which may require both pushing and pulling. Expect to pay $450 to $1200 for a sturdy machine.

How good is the workout? Excellent. And that's not surprising, considering research coming out of Scandinavia that found that cross-country skiers have the highest cardiovascular capacity of all endurance athletes. Yet for some the workout doesn't seem as hard as a bicycle (unless it is a dual-action arm and leg machine) or stair climber session. One reason is that the workload is divided among all the muscle groups of the body rather than being borne by just one group, as with a stair climber. Also, you can adjust the lower and upper body resistance separately on a cross-country skier to compensate for differences in strength.

Consider the cross-country ski workout even if you're involved in other sports. Because it works all the muscles of the body, cross-country skiing is used to complement many sports. Runners, in particular, often use skiers and stationary bicycles for cross-training in bad weather, or as a low-impact way to increase mileage when training for a marathon.

# HOW SKI MACHINES WORK

Because cross-country machines must accommodate a physical motion that would normally result in forward travel, the novice will tend to feel off balance and insecure at first. All cross-country machines induce this feeling of insecurity to some degree, at least in part because the most efficient posture for skiing is a slight forward lean. Some machines have a padded hip rest to keep you properly positioned; with the others, you maintain your balance by holding onto the poles.

Once on board, your job is to move one leg forward, hesitate, then push smoothly backward as you move the other leg forward. Meanwhile, work your poles in an alternating forward and backward motion, keeping your right arm in sync with your left leg, and vice versa. Hold your arms out fairly straight, and use your triceps to drive each hand down and back. Because your heels never actually strike the boards, you'll feel almost no stress on your knees and lower body.

## INDEPENDENT MODELS

All cross-country machines fall into two main categories according to whether the movement of the skis is independent or dependent. The first modern indoor ski machine introduced by NordicTrack in 1975 was an independent model. On these machines, the footpads move independently of each other, providing resistance only in the kick, or pushback, phase. A flywheel and belt mechanism provides smooth, continuous resistance, while a nylon-cord-and-pulley system provides resistance to the upper body. The machines do an adequate job of simulating the kick-and-glide motion of outdoor skiing, but they can be difficult to master.

The NordicTrack Achiever, at approximately $770, is made of wood and features elevated legs (for an uphill effect). By using the calibrated resistance settings on the upper and lower body exercises, you can accurately measure, in pounds or kilograms, the resistance working against your muscles.

The Precor 515E is made of aluminum and features a freewheel system, separate arm and leg adjustments, electronic monitors, and elevated legs. It sells for about $750 and is available in most fitness retail stores.

Manufacturers of independent machines admit there is a small learning curve for using their machine but claim that most well-coordinated individuals can be up and gliding in just a few hours.

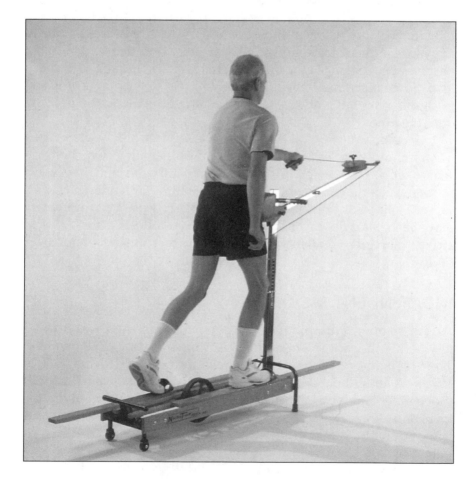

Because both the ski slats and arm pulleys have variable resistance settings and can be used independently of each other, beginning skiers can learn one skill first and then the other before putting the two together. Start by getting accustomed to the lower body motion by holding onto the hip rest (some models have handles for beginners), and later incorporate the hand cables or poles.

## DEPENDENT MODELS

In 1982, the first dependent skiers appeared on the market. On these machines, the footpads are linked by cables so that when one ski slides forward, the other automatically slides back, providing

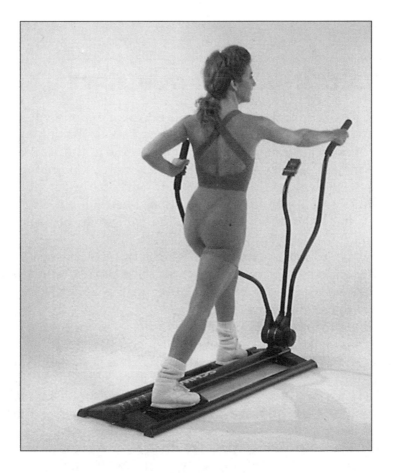

resistance in both directions. Although these machines can be mastered by even the most coordination-challenged exercisers, they do not provide as good an overall workout as an independent machine and don't come close to replicating the action of skiing on snow. If you cross-country ski on outdoor trails during the winter, the independent skier is the only way to go.

The Fitness Master FM 360i for about $700 is the best dependent skier on the market with an elaborate electronics panel. What makes the FM 360i unique, however, is its patented video interface. When you ski in place in front of your VCR and TV, an electronic eye on the control panel reads light signals off a specially encoded videotape containing cross-country footage and increases and decreases the resistance according to the terrain of the trail.

# SELECTING A SKI MACHINE

What type of machine best fits your needs: independent or dependent? If indoor skiing is new to you, spend about 15 minutes on each type of skier to learn the basic gliding motion of the arms and legs. Once mastered, the movements will become second nature, and if you have roller-skated or ice-skated, it will come much quicker. The shuffling and upper body motion should feel smooth. The poles or pulley cord should allow your arms full range of back-to-front motion.

Truly coordination-challenged? Check out the cheaper, easier-to-use dependent skiers. But before you buy, be aware that independent skiers give a superior workout and most people can eventually master the correct movement.

Make sure the height of the hip rest adjusts, as well as the height of the poles or lengths of the pulley cord, and that the tension on the poles and pulley is adjustable. The hip rest is designed to help you keep your balance, not to be leaned on forcefully during skiing.

The speed (resistance) and incline adjustment knobs should be easy to reach and adjust. Select a machine with feedback features you desire, such as heart rate, calories burned, and so on.

Most machines take up a lot of room. If floor space is at a premium, buy a machine that folds up easily for quick storage.

# WORKOUTS

Few of us do much skiing in our daily lives, so it is important to start slowly. Keep the resistance setting low at first. Beginners might want to start with 10- to 15-minute sessions that alternate 2 minutes of skiing with 30 seconds of rest. As you get stronger and more efficient, increase the duration and resistance gradually.

When the skiing action begins to feel routine, you can vary your program by adding sprints and intervals to your workouts. During sprints and interval training, you will be stressing your anaerobic energy system. Variety is essential to your training schedule and will improve your overall performance on the skier. Here are some ways to add power and variety to your workouts:

- Try pulling harder for 10 arm swings once every 2 to 3 minutes.

- Alternate three 5- to 6-minute periods of high-intensity skiing with three 3-minute periods of low-intensity skiing. Advanced skiers can increase the time and intensity of their workouts.

- Alternate 1 minute of all-out sprinting with 1 minute of easy skiing for a total of 20 minutes.

- Lengthen the periods of rest and make the sprints more intense; for example, 90 seconds to 2 minutes going all out followed by 3 minutes of easy skiing.

- If your goal is to lose weight, ski at an easy to moderate intensity for longer periods of time.

- In addition to the above workouts and those listed below, you can design workouts similar to those described for other pieces of equipment in the previous chapters.

## SONG REPEATS

Make a tape of your favorite psych-up tunes. Ski going all out for one song, then ease up through the next one. You can even choreograph a tape to include the right rhythms for warm-up and cool-down. Because you get a lot of rest during the slower songs, try to work on your technique and rhythm during them.

## HIGH-LOW WORKOUT

This endurance workout will vary your skiing technique and emphasize different muscle groups.

Warm up at an easy pace for 5 minutes.

For the next 5 minutes, increase the speed a little and take smooth strides.

For the next 5 minutes, increase the resistance on the arm pulley.

For the next 5 minutes, return to the settings of the first 5 minutes.

For 3 to 5 minutes, increase the resistance on the footpads.

Recover for 3 to 5 minutes at a slow to moderate rate and reduce the resistance.

For the next 5 minutes, increase the resistance on both the arm pulley and the footpads.

Cool down for 5 minutes at an easier resistance setting.

## TRAIL SKIING

This workout simulates a short race or a hard workout on back-country trails.

**Warm-up:** 5 to 10 minutes at an easy pace; heart rate at 50 to 60 percent of maximum.

**Steady-State Workout:** 20 to 30 minutes; heart rate in the 65 to 80 percent range.

**Intervals:** Increase tension on the skis and poles to simulate uphills. Alternate 30 seconds of uphill skiing with 30 seconds of downhill (recovery) for a total of 20 to 30 minutes. Vary the times as your fitness improves. Elevate your heart rate to 85 to 90 percent of maximum on the uphills.

**Cool-down:** 5 to 10 minutes of easy skiing, or until your heart rate falls below 55 percent of maximum.

## THE 10- TO 2-MINUTE DESCENDING LADDER

After a good warm-up, start with a 10-minute hard effort followed by 2 minutes of easy skiing for recovery. The next set should be 8 minutes hard, 2 minutes easy. Each hard set decreases in time by 2 minutes but increases slightly in intensity. The easy set remains the same. Vary the intensity of your arm and leg movements to add variety to the hard segments. The workout ends after you complete the 2-minute hard, 2-minute easy set.

## ✔ INJURY PREVENTION

Always warm up and stretch before your aerobic session.

Keep small children and pets away from moving parts of the exerciser while in use.

Don't let either of your feet slide in front of the stomach pad. This puts undue pressure on your knees.

Lift your heels while your feet are going back, and always keep your knees slightly bent.

Cool down and stretch after a hard session.

# LET IT SLIDE

Many Nordic skiers use cross-country machines, although more for conditioning than for maintaining or improving form. The machine's motion lacks the forward glide skiers get on snow, and its back-and-forth motion doesn't match the skating motion most cross-country skiers now use. So what started as a training device about 20 years ago has evolved into a conditioning machine—and one of the best around. Get on one for a half hour and you'll get a challenging aerobic workout without jarring your joints or back.

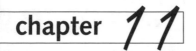

# Eating Right

## Jacqueline R. Berning, PhD, RD

Over the past 10 years, nutrition research as well as nutrition education have become a priority for many Americans. Today we recognize that a lack of nutrition knowledge and poor eating habits can contribute to poor fitness, low energy stores, and the development of lifestyle diseases such as heart disease, cancer, and diabetes. The time has come to start making wise food choices and commit to a fitness program.

The study of nutrition is a relative newcomer in the field of science. Only in the last 100 years or so have researchers begun to understand that nutrients found in food are needed for growth and health. Today we spend billions each year investigating the many aspects of nutrition, a science that encompasses the study not only of vitamins and minerals but also subjects as diverse as alcohol consumption, exercise, weight loss, and other nutrition-related fields.

At the same time, we are finding that, to some extent, we really are what we eat. Consumers are more confused than ever about how to translate the steady stream of new findings related to nutrition and fitness. Each new study that hits the media raises new concerns. Is caffeine bad for me? Should I be taking supplements? How much fat should I be eating? What foods should I be consuming to exercise more efficiently? Will certain foods make me more fit? How can I lose weight and keep it off?

# WHY WE EAT THE FOODS WE DO

Why are we so tempted by foods that have a high fat content and very few nutrients? What triggers our eating behaviors? Why do we like certain foods?

Many factors influence our food choices, including hunger, habit, economics, marketing, availability, convenience, nutritional value, and psychological effects, to name just a few. One reason we choose certain foods is taste preference. Most of us like the taste of sugar and salt, and as a result we tend to eat too many sweets and salty foods, especially snacks. We also like foods that have happy associations—such as those we eat at family gatherings or on holidays, or those someone who loved us gave us as children. By the same token, we avoid certain foods because of negative associations—such as foods we ate just before catching the flu, or foods we were forced to eat as young children, or foods associated with times of tragedy.

Social pressure has a very powerful influence on food choices. Many of us have been programmed to feel that it's rude not to accept food in certain social situations, or that our friends will be offended if we don't go out for pizza and beer with them. Social pressure is at work in every culture and every social circle. We've all felt the pressure of being forced to eat at office celebrations, family gatherings (especially at our mother-in-law's house), and other social events.

Availability, convenience, and economics also play a role in food selection. You cannot eat foods that are not available, or that you cannot afford, and you're more likely to choose foods that are convenient over ones that are difficult to prepare (such as popping a frozen pizza in the oven versus preparing a meal from scratch).

Food behavior is also related to psychological needs, such as an infant's association of food with parental love. Some people respond to stress—positive or negative—by eating; others may use food to ward off loneliness, boredom, or anxiety.

As you can see, of the variety of reasons for choosing foods, few of them have to do with nutritional value. So, how do you go about selecting foods that have more nutrients than calories (are nutrient dense) so that you can achieve optimal health and fitness? To do so successfully, you need to learn what nutrients the body needs and what foods supply them.

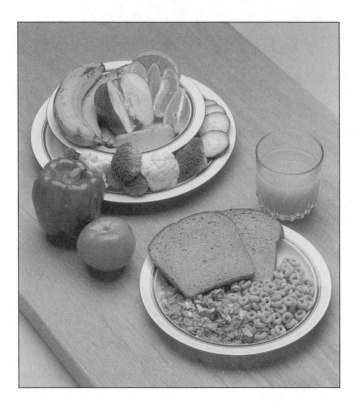

# ESSENTIAL NUTRIENTS

Nutrients are life-sustaining substances obtained from food. They work together to supply us with energy to perform on and off the job as well as to maintain our health. Protein, carbohydrate, fat, vitamins, minerals, and water are the six major classes of nutrients. Table 11.1 lists the nutrient classes and their major functions. The amounts of nutrients your body needs vary widely from one nutrient to another; however there are standards for making sure that you receive enough nutrients to sustain a healthy and active lifestyle.

## RECOMMENDED NUTRIENT INTAKES

Assuming you are a normal, healthy adult of average size who engages in physical activity, you need to consume the following amounts of nutrients daily to remain in optimal health:

**Table 11.1    The Six Classes of Nutrients and Their Major Functions**

| Nutrient | Function |
|---|---|
| Protein | • Build and repair body tissue<br>• Major component of enzymes, hormones, and antibodies |
| Carbohydrate | • Provide a major source of fuel to the body<br>• Provide dietary fibers |
| Fat | • Chief storage form of energy in the body<br>• Insulate and protect vital organs<br>• Provide fat-soluble vitamins |
| Vitamins | • Help promote and regulate various chemical reactions and bodily processes<br>• Do not yield energy themselves but participate in releasing energy from food |
| Minerals | • Enable enzymes to function<br>• A component of hormones<br>• A part of bone and nerve impulses |
| Water | • Enables chemical reactions to occur<br>• About 60% of the body is composed of water<br>• Essential for life as we cannot store it or conserve it |

- Protein—approximately 50-70 grams, depending on body size, or 12-20 percent of calorie intake from protein.

- Carbohydrate—minimum 125 grams, optimal 350-400 grams, or 55-60 percent of calorie intake from carbohydrates.

- Fat—approximately 30-65 grams, depending on caloric consumption, or 25-30 percent of calorie intake from fat.

- Vitamins—specific amounts are listed in the Recommended Dietary Allowances (RDAs); see Table 11.2.

- Minerals—specific amounts are listed in the RDAs; see Table 11.2.

- Water—2 to 3 quarts per day.

The Recommended Dietary Allowances are nutrient recommendations that meet the needs of essentially all people of similar age and gender. Established by the Food and Nutrition Board of the National Academy of Sciences, they are a guide for estimating your nutritional needs. RDAs are expressed as an optimal amount with upper and lower limits—meaning that too little is not good and too much may also present problems. Many Americans believe that if a little is good, more has got to be better. However, in nutrition, that kind of thinking may lead to toxicities, especially with some fat-soluble vitamins.

The RDAs are to be used as a guide . . . a ballpark figure, if you will. Just because you only take in 40 mg of Vitamin C on a particular day does not mean that the next day you'll come down with scurvy (the disease caused by Vitamin C deficiency). Symptoms of nutritional deficiencies may be subtle and develop slowly. It takes a long time to detect problems. If you suspect that your diet is not nutritious enough, don't wait for warning signs to develop. Start eating foods the meet your RDA for all listed nutrients rather than risk developing health problems due to poor nutrition.

## CARBOHYDRATES

Carbohydrate is the most important, and least abundant, nutrient for working muscles. Adequate amounts of carbohydrate are essential for muscular performance as well as for brain and central nervous system function. The principal functions of carbohydrates are to:

- serve as a primary energy source for working muscles,
- ensure that the brain and nervous system function properly, and
- help the body use fat more efficiently.

Stored carbohydrates (glycogen) are the primary fuel for exercise. If you are having a hard time maintaining normal workout intensities, it may indicate that you have inadequate muscle carbohydrate or glycogen levels. Unless adequate glycogen levels are restored, your exercise will continue to deteriorate to the point where even an easy workout will cause fatigue.

At lease 55 percent of daily calorie consumption should be from carbohydrates. For Americans, about 45 percent of our daily calorie consumption is from carbohydrates, much of it in the form of simple carbohydrates or sugars rather than complex carbohydrates such as breads, cereals, pasta, and rice. Table 11.3 lists good sources of carbohydrates, including gram amounts. Remember, if you need a boost of energy or are hungry and want something to eat, try a food that is rich in carbohydrates and low in fat.

## Table 11.2 Recommended Dietary Allowances

| Category | Age | Weight (lb) | Height (in) | Protein (g) | Fat-soluble vitamins | | | | Water-soluble vitamins | | |
|---|---|---|---|---|---|---|---|---|---|---|---|
| | | | | | Vitamin A (mcg RE)[a] | Vitamin D (mcg) | Vitamin E (mg)[b] | Vitamin K (mcg) | Vitamin C (mg) | Thiamin (mg) | Riboflavin (mg) |
| Males | 15-18 | 145 | 69 | 59 | 1,000 | 10 | 10 | 65 | 60 | 1.5 | 1.8 |
| | 19-24 | 160 | 70 | 58 | 1,000 | 10 | 10 | 70 | 60 | 1.5 | 1.7 |
| | 25-50 | 174 | 70 | 63 | 1,000 | 5 | 10 | 80 | 60 | 1.5 | 1.7 |
| | 51+ | 170 | 68 | 63 | 1,000 | 5 | 10 | 80 | 60 | 1.2 | 1.4 |
| Females | 15-18 | 120 | 64 | 44 | 800 | 10 | 8 | 55 | 60 | 1.1 | 1.3 |
| | 19-24 | 128 | 65 | 46 | 800 | 10 | 8 | 60 | 60 | 1.1 | 1.3 |
| | 25-50 | 138 | 64 | 50 | 800 | 5 | 8 | 65 | 60 | 1.1 | 1.3 |
| | 51+ | 143 | 63 | 50 | 800 | 5 | 8 | 65 | 60 | 1.0 | 1.2 |

(continued)

**Table 11.2**   Recommended Dietary Allowances *(continued)*

| Category | Age | Water-soluble vitamins | | | | Minerals | | | | | | |
|---|---|---|---|---|---|---|---|---|---|---|---|---|
| | | Niacin (mg) | Vitamin B$_6$ (mg) | Folate (mcg) | Vitamin B$_{12}$ (mcg) | Calcium (mg) | Phos-phorus (mg) | Magne-sium (mg) | Iron (mg) | Zinc (mg) | Iodine (mcg) | Selenium (mcg) |
| Males | 15-18 | 20 | 2.0 | 200 | 2.0 | 1,200 | 1,200 | 400 | 12 | 15 | 150 | 50 |
| | 19-24 | 19 | 2.0 | 200 | 2.0 | 1,200 | 1,200 | 350 | 10 | 15 | 150 | 70 |
| | 25-50 | 19 | 2.0 | 200 | 2.0 | 800 | 800 | 350 | 10 | 15 | 150 | 70 |
| | 51+ | 15 | 2.0 | 200 | 2.0 | 800 | 800 | 350 | 10 | 15 | 150 | 70 |
| Females | 15-18 | 15 | 1.5 | 180 | 2.0 | 1,200 | 1,200 | 300 | 15 | 12 | 150 | 70 |
| | 19-24 | 15 | 1.6 | 180 | 2.0 | 1,200 | 1,200 | 280 | 15 | 12 | 150 | 55 |
| | 25-50 | 15 | 1.6 | 180 | 2.0 | 800 | 800 | 280 | 15 | 12 | 150 | 55 |
| | 51+ | 13 | 1.6 | 180 | 2.0 | 800 | 800 | 280 | 10 | 12 | 150 | 55 |

[a]mcg - microgram = 1/1,000,000th gram; RE - retinol equivalent = 1 mcg retinol or 6 mcg beta-carotene
[b]mg - milligram = 1/1,000th gram

Source: Food and Nutrition Board, National Academy of Sciences—National Research Council Recommended Dietary Allowances, Revised 1989. Recommended Dietary Allowances (RDAs) are established by the National Research Council of the National Academy of Sciences and published by the Government. The RDA for any given nutrient represents the amount considered "adequate to meet the known nutrient needs of practically all healthy persons."

**Table 11.3  Foods Listed by Groups with Carbohydrate Content**

| Food group | Serving | Calories | Carbo-hydrate (g) | Food group | Serving | Calories | Carbo-hydrate (g) |
|---|---|---|---|---|---|---|---|
| **Milk** | | | | Frozen yogurt (low-fat) | 1 cup | 220 | 34 |
| Low-fat milk (2%) | 1 cup/8 oz. | 121 | 12 | Fruit-flavored yogurt (low-fat) | 1 cup | 225 | 43 |
| Skim milk | 1 cup | 86 | 12 | | | | |
| Chocolate milk | 1 cup | 208 | 26 | | | | |
| Pudding (any flavor) | 1/2 cup | 161 | 30 | | | | |
| | | | | Grapes | 1 cup | 58 | 16 |
| **Fruit** | | | | Grape juice | 1 cup | 96 | 23 |
| Apple | 1 medium | 81 | 21 | Orange | 1 medium | 65 | 16 |
| Apple juice | 1 cup | 111 | 28 | Orange juice | 1 cup | 112 | 26 |
| Applesauce | 1 cup | 194 | 52 | Pear | 1 medium | 98 | 25 |
| Banana | 1 medium | 105 | 27 | Pineapple | 1 cup | 77 | 19 |
| Cantaloupe | 1 cup | 57 | 13 | Prunes (dried) | 10 | 201 | 53 |
| Cherries (raw) | 10 | 49 | 11 | Raisins | 2/3 cup | 300 | 79 |
| Cranberry juice cocktail | 1 cup | 147 | 37 | Raspberries | 1 cup | 61 | 14 |
| Dates (dried) | 10 | 228 | 61 | Strawberries | 1 cup | 45 | 11 |
| Fruit cocktail (in own juice) | 1/2 cup | 56 | 15 | Watermelon | 1 cup | 50 | 12 |
| Fruit roll-ups | 1 roll | 50 | 12 | | | | |

*(continued)*

**Table 11.3   Foods Listed by Groups with Carbohydrate Content** (*continued*)

| Food group | Serving | Calories | Carbo-hydrate (g) | Food group | Serving | Calories | Carbo-hydrate (g) |
|---|---|---|---|---|---|---|---|
| **Vegetable** | | | | | | | |
| Black-eyed peas | 1/2 cup | 99 | 78 | Pinto beans | 1 cup | 235 | 44 |
| Carrots | 1/2 cup | 31 | 7 | Potato | 1 large | 139 | 32 |
| Corn | 1/2 cup | 88 | 21 | Refried beans | 1 cup | 270 | 47 |
| Garbanzo beans (chickpeas) | 1 cup | 269 | 45 | Sweet potato | 1 large | 118 | 28 |
| | | | | Three-bean salad | 1/2 cup | 90 | 20 |
| Lima beans | 1 cup | 217 | 39 | Water chestnuts | 1/2 cup | 66 | 15 |
| Navy beans | 1 cup | 259 | 48 | White beans | 1 cup | 249 | 45 |
| Peas (green) | 1/2 cup | 63 | 12 | | | | |
| **Grain** | | | | | | | |
| Bagel | 1 | 163 | 31 | Graham crackers | 2 squares | 63 | 11 |
| Biscuit | 1 | 103 | 13 | Saltines | 5 crackers | 60 | 10 |
| White bread | 1 slice | 61 | 12 | Triscuit crackers | 3 crackers | 60 | 10 |
| Whole wheat bread | 1 slice | 61 | 11 | Pancakes | 1 | 61 | 9 |
| Breadsticks | 2 sticks | 77 | 15 | Waffles | 1 | 130 | 17 |
| Cornbread | 1 square | 178 | 28 | Rice | 1 cup | 206 | 50 |
| Cereal (ready-to-eat) | 1 cup | 110 | 24 | Rice (brown) | 1 cup | 232 | 50 |
| Cream of Wheat | 3/4 cup | 96 | 20 | Hamburger bun | 1 | 119 | 21 |
| Malt-O-Meal | 3/4 cup | 92 | 19 | Hot dog bun | 1 | 119 | 21 |
| Flavored oatmeal (instant) | 1 packet | 110 | 25 | Noodles (spaghetti) | 1 cup | 159 | 34 |
| | | | | Flour tortilla | 1 | 95 | 17 |
| GatorLode™ | 11.6 oz | 280 | 70 | | | | |
| GatorPro™ | 11 oz | 360 | 59 | | | | |

Adapted from *Sports Nutrition in the 90s*, by Jacqueline Berning and Suzanne Nelson Steen, pp. 40–41. Copyright 1991 Aspen Publishers, Inc.

# PROTEIN

The principal role of dietary protein is to build and repair body tissues, including muscles, ligaments, and tendons. Contrary to popular belief, protein is not a primary source of energy, except when you don't consume enough calories or carbohydrates. If you fail to eat enough calories, protein is broken down and used as an energy source instead of being used for its intended job of tissue building.

Protein is made up of amino acids. When protein foods are eaten, these amino acids are absorbed and used to form muscle, hemoglobin, enzymes, and hormones. Whenever you consume more protein than your body can use, the excess amino acids are stored as fat. Research suggests that an adult needs about 0.8-1.0 grams of protein per kilogram of body weight. For example, a 45-year-old man who weighs 155 pounds needs 56-70 grams of protein per day.

The typical American diet supplies about 1.5 grams of protein per kilogram of body weight, which is adequate for most active adults to support growth and muscle development. Sedentary adults need only about 0.8 grams of protein per kilogram of body weight each day, while adolescents need slightly more (1.0 grams per kilogram of body weight).

To determine your own protein requirement use the following equation:

weight in pounds _____
$\div$ 2.2 = _____ (your weight in kilograms)

Your weight in kilograms _____
$\times$ 0.8 = _____ grams of protein per day.

For example, the daily protein requirement for a sedentary person who weighs 165 pounds would be:

165 pounds $\div$ 2.2 = 76 kilograms
$\times$ 0.8 = 60 grams of protein per day.

To determine the amount of protein in food, use the following as a guide:

- 8 grams of protein per cup of milk, yogurt, or any serving of dairy products
- 8 grams of protein per ounce of cheese

- 7 grams of protein per ounce of meat (beef, chicken, fish)
- 3 grams of protein per serving of bread or grains (1 slice of bread, 1/2 cup of rice, 1/2 cup of pasta)

Table 11.4 lists the specific amounts of protein in some common protein-rich foods.

# THE FOOD GUIDE PYRAMID

Although the RDAs list specific amounts of nutrients to consume, they make only general statements about energy (calorie intake) and

## Table 11.4    Protein Amounts Found in Common Foods

| Food | Portion size | Protein (g) |
| --- | --- | --- |
| **Animal sources** | | |
| Milk (skim, 2%, whole) | 1 cup | 8 |
| Yogurt (nonfat, low-fat) | 1 cup | 8 |
| Cheese (any variety) | 1 oz | 8 |
| Lean hamburger patty | 3 oz | 26 |
| Egg/egg white | 1 | 7 |
| Lean steak | 3 oz | 21 |
| Lean pork chop | 3 oz | 21 |
| Chicken breast | 3.5 oz | 30 |
| Turkey | 3 oz | 21 |
| Taco | 1 | 11 |
| Pizza | 2 slices | 32 |
| Tuna | 3 oz | 24 |
| **Plant sources** | | |
| Peanut butter | 1 T | 4 |
| Whole wheat bread | 1 slice | 3 |
| Pasta | 1 cup | 4 |
| Almonds | 12-15 | 3 |
| Beans | 1/2 cup | 7 |
| Cereal | 1/2 cup | 3 |

Any of the animal proteins will provide complete protein. Plant sources of protein have one or more amino acids missing. Combining two plant sources will provide complete proteins; for example, a peanut butter sandwich on whole wheat bread.
Data from *Food Values of Portions Commonly Used* (15th ed.) by J.A. Pennington, Harper & Row, 1989.

do little to protect you from excess fat, sugar, salt, cholesterol, and alcohol in your diet. Today health specialists are just as concerned about moderation in the diet as they are about consuming too few or too many nutrients. For that reason, the U.S. Department of Agriculture (USDA) recently developed the Food Guide Pyramid, a guide to daily food choices comprising six food groups. Foods grouped together are similar in calorie and nutrient content. The major differences between the Food Guide Pyramid and the old four food groups are that fruits and vegetables are classified into their own separate groups and the recommended number of servings from those groups is increased from 4 to 9 per day. Another difference is that the recommended number of servings from the grain group is increased from 4 per day to 6 to 11 per day to provide the bulk of dietary intake from carbohydrate while limiting fat. This is reflected in the placement of food groups in the pyramid—grains, fruits, and vegetables form the foundation, and although the meat and dairy groups are still essential in the diet, they play a lesser role.

The Food Guide Pyramid is a practical way to turn the RDAs into food choices. By eating a balanced variety of foods each day from the food groups listed in the pyramid, you will get all the essential

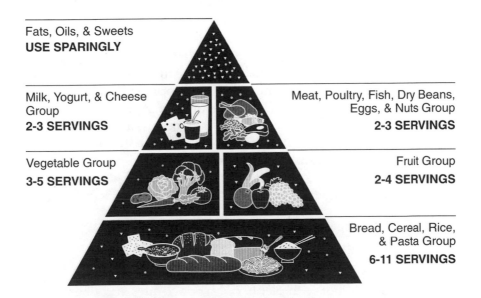

Food Guide Pyramid.
From the U.S. Department of Agriculture/U.S. Department of Health and Human Services.

nutrients to reach and maintain a desirable weight. The minimum number of servings in each food group provide approximately 1,600 to 1,800 calories. Table 11.5 summarizes the recommended servings per day, the major nutrient contributions, and the serving sizes of sample foods from each group in the Food Guide Pyramid. Below are other points to keep in mind when you use the Food Guide Pyramid:

1. The guide does not apply to infants or to children under 2 years of age.

2. No one food provides all the essential nutrients, and therefore you must eat a wide variety of foods from each group.

3. Variety is the key to the plan. Variety is guaranteed by choosing foods from all groups and selecting different foods within each group.

Remember, the key to nutrition is to consume a wide variety of foods from each of the food groups within the food pyramid and to moderate your intake of calories from fat and sugar.

# DIETARY GUIDELINES

During the late 70s and early 80s, national health agencies and scientific councils developed guidelines to address the more recently identified dietary imbalances that contribute to the leading causes of death in the United States and other developing countries. In response to these concerns, the U.S. Department of Agriculture and the Department of Health and Human Services issued the Dietary Guidelines, seven principles that all Americans should know to reduce their risk of diet-related diseases such as cancer, heart disease, diabetes, hypertension, and obesity, to name just a few.

The Dietary Guidelines for Americans recommend:

1. choosing a wide variety of foods;

2. achieving and maintaining a healthy weight;

3. choosing a diet low in fat, saturated fat, and cholesterol;

4. choosing a diet with plenty of carbohydrates and fiber;

5. using sugar in moderation;

## Table 11.5  The Food Guide Pyramid—A Summary

| Food group | Serving | Major contributions | Food and serving size |
|---|---|---|---|
| Milk, yogurt, cheese | 2-3 adults 3-4 children, teens, pregnant or lactating women | Calcium Carbohydrate Riboflavin Protein Zinc Potassium | 1 cup milk 1-1/2 oz of cheese 1 cup yogurt 2 cups cottage cheese 1 cup pudding |
| Meat, poultry, fish, dry beans, eggs, nuts | 2-3 | Protein Niacin Iron Vitamin $B_6$ Zinc Thiamin Vitamin $B_{12}$ | 2-3 oz meat, poultry, or fish 1-1/2 cups beans 2 T peanut butter 2 eggs 1/2-1 cup nuts |
| Fruits | 2-4 | Carbohydrate Vitamin C Fiber | 1/4 cup dried fruit 1/2 cup cooked fruit 3/4 cup juice 1 whole piece of fruit |
| Vegetables | 3-5 | Carbohydrate Vitamin A Vitamin C Folate Magnesium Dietary fiber | 1/2 cup raw or cooked 1 cup leafy greens 1/2 cup vegetable juice |
| Bread, cereals, rice, pasta | 6-11 | Carbohydrate Thiamin Riboflavin Iron Niacin Folate Magnesium Fiber Zinc | 1 slice of bread 1 oz of ready-to-eat cereal 1/2-3/4 cup cooked cereal, pasta, or rice |
| Fats, oils, sweets | | Foods from this group should not replace any from the other groups. Amounts consumed should be determined by individual energy needs. | |

Data from the U.S. Department of Agriculture/U.S. Department of Health and Human Services.

6. using sodium in moderation; and

7. if you drink alcohol, doing so in moderation.

Specifically, experts recommend that you reduce your intake of all fats to no more than 30 percent of total calories consumed. The current consumption of fat in this country is around 34 percent of daily calorie intake. Saturated fat should provide no more than 10 percent of calorie intake, and cholesterol should not exceed 300 milligrams daily. To achieve this, nutritionists suggest that we substitute additional carbohydrates and *unsaturated* fats for saturated fats. Obvious sources of fat include butter, margarine, shortening, and oils. But fats are also present in food products such as marbled meats, poultry skin, whole milk, cheese, ice cream, nuts, peanut butter, salad dressing, many snack foods, and most bakery products. Fried foods are also high in fats. Foods that are low in fat include starchy or complex carbohydrates such as breads, pasta, potatoes, rice, and beans. Other low-fat foods include fruits, vegetables, skim milk, low-fat yogurt, and fish. To lower the fat in your diet, try the simple substitutes found in Table 11.6 (p. 198). To find out how much fat you are eating, answer the questions in the How Do You Score on Fat? worksheet.

# WEIGHT CONTROL

Caloric requirements differ for everyone and are determined by age, sex, weight, and physical activity. Weight is a matter of balance between caloric intake and caloric expenditure. Your body weight will change when there is an imbalance between caloric intake and caloric expenditure in the form of exercise. To lose weight, energy output must be greater than energy intake. In short, to lose weight, you must eat less or exercise more, or both.

## PROPER WEIGHT LOSS TECHNIQUES

To lose 1 pound, you would either have to run about 35 miles or eat 3,500 fewer calories. Obviously, it would be difficult to do either in a short time. To put weight loss in perspective, use the formula below:

3,500 calories ÷ 7 days per week = 500 calories per day.

# HOW DO YOU SCORE ON FAT?

Do the foods you eat provide more fat than is good for you? Answer the questions below, then see how your diet stacks up.

| How often do you eat: | 1-2 times a week | 3-5 times a week | Almost daily |
| --- | --- | --- | --- |
| Fried or breaded foods? | | | |
| Fatty meats such as bacon, sausage, luncheon meats, and heavily marbled steaks and roasts? | | | |
| Whole milk, high-fat cheeses, and ice cream? | | | |
| High-fat desserts such as pies, pastries, and rich cakes? | | | |
| Sauces and gravies? | | | |
| Oily salad dressings and mayonnaise? | | | |
| Whipped cream, table cream, sour cream, and cream cheese? | | | |
| Butter or margarine on vegetables, dinner rolls, bread, and toast? | | | |

Take a look at your answers. If there are several responses in the last two columns, you may have a high fat intake. Is it time to cut back on foods high in fat?

Adapted from USDA Home and Garden Bulletin No. 232-1, Washington D.C. Government Printing Office, April, 1986.

### Table 11.6   Fat Substitutions

| Instead of: | Try: |
| --- | --- |
| • Whole milk | Skim milk |
| • Cheddar, Jack, or Swiss cheese | Part-skim mozzarella, string, or low-fat cottage cheese, other cheeses that contain less than 5 g of fat per ounce |
| • Ice cream | Ice milk or low-fat/nonfat frozen yogurt |
| • Butter or margarine | Jam, yogurt, ricotta cheese, light or nonfat cream cheese |
| • Sour cream | Low-fat yogurt, light sour cream, blender-whipped cottage cheese dressing |
| • Bacon | Canadian bacon or bacon bits |
| • Ground beef | Extra lean ground beef or ground turkey |
| • Fried chicken | Baked chicken without the skin |
| • Doughnuts and pastries | Bagels, whole-grain breads, homemade breads, muffins, or quick breads |
| • Apple pie | Baked or raw apple |
| • Chocolate candy or bars | Jelly beans, hard candy, licorice |
| • Cookies, cakes, brownies | Vanilla wafers, gingersnaps, graham crackers, fig bars |

Put simply, to lose 1 pound per week you would need to eat 500 fewer calories per day.  By burning 250 calories each day through exercise, you only need to reduce your calorie intake by 250 per day to still achieve a weight loss of 1 pound per week. What's more, it would be a healthier, more balanced weight loss.

A daily caloric deficit can range from 250 to 500 calories per day (depending on how active you are), but your average weight loss should not exceed 2 pounds per week. This mild caloric restriction results in a manageable loss of water, electrolytes, minerals, and lean body tissue and is less likely to cause malnutrition. It is recommended that any weight loss regimen include exercise.

Weight loss is most successful when diet and exercise are combined to create a calorie deficit that results in lasting weight loss. Caloric intake can be decreased by eating fewer calories from foods that are calorie dense, such as those that contain high amounts of sugar, fat, and alcohol. Eating habits can also be improved by eating regular

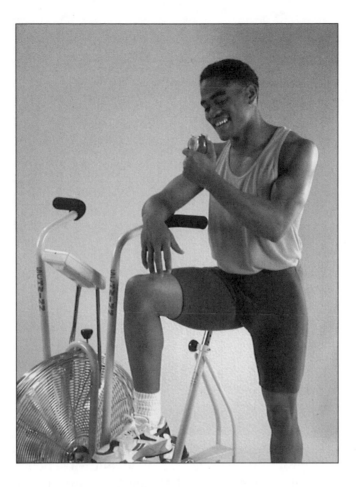

meals. Individuals who eat two or three large meals a day will have more difficulty losing weight than individuals who eat the same amount of calories in five or six meals throughout the day. Also, eating smaller, more frequent meals spreads the energy intake evenly throughout the day, making energy readily available for exercise. Table 11.7 gives some examples of exercise activities and their caloric costs.

## WHY NOT CRASH DIET?

It is human nature to search for a quick way to lose weight. It may have taken a year to put on that excess 10 pounds, but we want it off in a week. Fad diets are popular because they promote rapid, temporary weight loss. But crash diets actually result in loss of lean

### Table 11.7 Exercise Activities and Their Caloric Expenditure

| Physical effort | Caloric expenditure (calories per min) | |
| --- | --- | --- |
| | Men | Women |
| Very light sleeping, lying, sitting, driving, standing | <2 | <1 |
| Light, slow walking, golf, shopping, trade work | 2.5-5.0 | 1.5-3.5 |
| Moderate, fast walking, cycling, tennis, dancing | 5.0-7.5 | 3.5-5.5 |
| Vigorous swimming, basketball, walking uphill with a load | 7.5-10.0 | 5.5-7.5 |
| Very vigorous running, climbing | 10.0-12.5 | 7.5-9.5 |
| Exhausting | >15.0 | >9.5 |

Adapted from Katch and McArdle (1993).

muscle mass, water, and stored energy, not excess body fat. As a result, individuals on such diets become fatigued early in the day and have a hard time finding the energy to work out. Most people regard the rapid weight loss as evidence that they are losing fat, when in fact their body fat stores are virtually untouched.

To lose weight safely and effectively, it is important to eat a variety of foods from each of the food groups found in the Food Guide Pyramid, consuming enough carbohydrate to fuel exercise and lowering fat consumption for calorie restriction, rather than following a restrictive diet.

## YO-YO DIETING

Chronic dieting and repeated weight loss followed by weight gain (yo-yo dieting) may increase the energy efficiency of the body. This means the body adapts to fewer calories. For example, after repeated yo-yo dieting, an individual who was able to lose weight eating 1,500 calories in the past may no longer lose weight eating that amount of calories. To lose weight, he or she may have to eat as few as 1,200 calories. The resistance to weight loss in yo-yo dieting (as well as fad dieting) is thought to be due to the body responding to these extremely low-calorie diets by lowering the rate at which it burns calories (metabolic rate) to fight off what it perceives to be starvation. Although there is controversy as to whether or not yo-yo dieting lowers metabolic rate, it may alter body composition, specifically increasing the proportion of body fat while lowering the proportion of lean muscle mass.

# THE GAME PLAN

Remember, nutrition is one of the key factors in an overall fitness program. Making sure that you are eating a wide variety of foods from each of the food groups and moderating your consumption of foods that are high in fat, sugar, and sodium will lower your risk for lifestyle diseases. This does not mean that you have to starve yourself, or that you can never eat your favorite foods again. On the contrary, combining a home fitness program and a nutritious diet will enable you to enjoy the best years of your life.

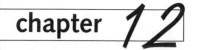

# Using Home Workouts for Fitness

**Wayne L. Westcott, PhD**

During the past several years, thousands of men and women have exercised in our Boston-area YMCA fitness center. Although it is a large facility with a wide variety of strength and endurance equipment, most of our members follow a very simple training format. Basically, they complete three 60-minute exercise sessions per week. Each session includes 20-25 minutes of strength exercise and 20-25 minutes of endurance exercise. The remaining time is divided between 5-10 minutes of warm-up activity and 5-10 minutes of cool-down activity.

The results of this sensible program of regular exercise have been very encouraging. After 2 months of training, the participants typically add 3 pounds of muscle and lose 9 pounds of fat, for a 12-pound improvement in their body composition and physical appearance. They also increase their muscular strength, cardiovascular endurance, and joint flexibility. In addition, they experience significant reductions in their resting blood pressure. Finally, they report major improvements in energy level, physical activity, and self-confidence.

Is it possible for you to attain similar exercise benefits from a home training program? Certainly, but you may need to follow a fairly structured program to maintain motivation until your exercise sessions become habitual. When you go to a fitness facility, you are in an exercise environment where everyone is working out. However, your home may not elicit the same activity patterns until you develop a regular exercise routine.

It is better to start small and systematically expand your exercise program than to start big and have to cut back your activity level due to overtraining or time constraints.

# STRENGTH TRAINING WORKOUTS

Strength training is one of the keys to physical fitness because your muscles are the engines of your body. Consequently, increasing your muscle strength is similar to driving an eight-cylinder car rather than a four-cylinder car. You have a greater muscular capacity to perform all kinds of physical activities.

Regardless of your present level of strength, you can select an appropriate resistance to safely and successfully develop your muscular fitness. Fortunately, young and old, males and females experience similar strength benefits from training in a sensible and systematic manner.

The guidelines for improving your strength fitness are relatively simple to understand and apply. According to the American College of Sports Medicine, a basic program of strength exercise should follow these training procedures:

1. Perform a minimum of 8 to 10 strength exercises involving the major muscle groups.

2. Train at least 2 days per week.

3. Perform a minimum of one set of strength exercises for each major muscle group.

4. Use a resistance that permits 8 to 12 repetitions to the point of near muscle fatigue.

5. Perform each repetition at a moderate to slow movement speed.

6. Perform each repetition through a full movement range.

7. Breathe continuously throughout each set of exercises.

You may choose to perform more than 8 to 10 exercises, do more than one set, and train more than twice a week. However, these recommendations provide an excellent starting point that should not overstress your musculoskeletal system, and from which you can progressively increase your training demands.

# BEGINNER PROGRAM

I recommend that you find an appropriate resistance for each exercise through trial and error procedures. Generally speaking, you should use a resistance that permits about 10 controlled repetitions per exercise set with a range of 8 to 12 repetitions. When you can complete 12 repetitions, you should increase the resistance by approximately 5 percent. For example, when you can perform 12 repetitions with 50 pounds, you should add 2.5 pounds.

Start with one set of each exercise, as this should provide a sufficient strength-building stimulus. However, you may perform two sets of each exercise after 2 weeks of training, and three sets after 4 weeks of training, if you desire. If you choose to do multiple exercise sets, you should rest about 2 minutes between sets.

You may want to begin with two training sessions per week, then progress to a 3-day-per-week training program as your strength fitness improves. Just be sure to schedule at least 48 hours of recovery and building time between each strength workout.

As you become accustomed to your strength program, you may periodically change your exercise resistance and training repetitions. For example, you may perform fewer repetitions (4-8) with high resistance or more repetitions (12-16) with low resistance. Just remember to perform every exercise set with proper training technique.

Let's look at two sample strength training programs for beginning exercisers. The first is performed on weight stack machines, and the second is done with free weights.

## Weight Stack Machines

Typical strength training protocols begin with exercises for the larger muscles of the legs, then progress to the muscles of the torso, arms, and midsection. Although you may prefer a different training sequence, the following exercise order should be productive. (See chapter 5 for a more complete description of these exercises.)

- Leg extensions for the quadriceps muscles in the front of the thigh.
- Prone or standing leg curls for the hamstrings muscles in the back of the thigh.
- Chest presses for the pectoral muscles in the front of the torso.
- Low rowing (also called seated rows) for the latissimus muscles in the back of the torso.
- Shoulder presses for the deltoid muscles in the upper torso.
- Arm curls for the biceps muscles in the front of the arm.
- Triceps extensions and triceps pushdowns for the triceps muscles in the back of the arm.
- Abdominal crunches for the abdominal muscles in the midsection.

## BEGINNING WEIGHT STACK MACHINE PROGRAM

| Monday, Wednesday, and Friday | Sets | Repetitions |
|---|---|---|
| Leg Extension | 1 | 8-12 |
| Leg Curl | 1 | 8-12 |
| Chest Press | 1 | 8-12 |
| Low Rowing | 1 | 8-12 |
| Shoulder Press | 1 | 8-12 |
| Arm Curl | 1 | 8-12 |
| Triceps Extension | 1 | 8-12 |
| Abdominal Crunches | 1 | 8-12 |

## Free Weights

Free-weight training is typically performed with barbells and dumbbells. If you are a novice with free weights, you should start out with dumbbells, because it is safer than barbell training. For example, failure to complete a barbell bench press may result in having a barbell perched across your chest. Also, a barbell bent row may place high stress on your lower back, whereas a dumbbell bent row allows you to support your torso weight with your non-exercising arm. The following dumbbell exercise program should be effective for strength-ening your major muscle groups.

- Barbell squats for the quadriceps and hamstrings muscles in the thigh.
- Dumbbell lunges for the quadriceps and hamstrings muscles in the thigh.
- Barbell bench presses for the pectoral muscles in the front of the torso.
- One-arm dumbbell rows for the latissimus muscles in the back of the torso.
- Dumbbell lateral raises for the deltoid muscles in the upper torso.
- Dumbbell arm curls for the biceps muscles in the front of the arm.
- Dumbbell triceps kickbacks for the triceps muscles in the back of the arm.
- Trunk curls for the abdominal muscles in the midsection.

## BEGINNING FREE-WEIGHT PROGRAM

| Monday, Wednesday, and Friday | Sets | Repetitions |
|---|---|---|
| Squat | 1 | 8-12 |
| Dumbbell Lunge | 1 | 8-12 |
| Bench Press | 1 | 8-12 |
| One-Arm Dumbbell Row | 1 | 8-12 |
| Dumbbell Lateral Raise | 1 | 8-12 |
| Dumbbell Arm Curl | 1 | 8-12 |
| Dumbbell Triceps Kickback | 1 | 8-12 |
| Trunk Curl | 1 | 8-12 |

## INTERMEDIATE PROGRAM

Whether you perform one, two, or three sets of strength exercises, at some point you will stop making progress and experience a strength plateau. The first thing to consider in overcoming a strength plateau is a change in your training exercises. Your muscles are very adaptable, and they may become so accustomed to a particular exercise that it no longer provides an effective training stimulus.

For example, if you are not improving in shoulder presses, you should try substituting lateral raises. Although both exercises target the deltoid muscles, the different movement patterns involve different muscle fiber activation and elicit different training responses.

The second thing to consider in overcoming a strength plateau is an increase in your training intensity. That is, making each set of exercises more productive by increasing the training demands. One means of achieving this objective is to extend your training set with a few (typically two to four) breakdown repetitions.

For example, you may complete 10 biceps curls with 30-pound dumbbells, but find your biceps muscles are too fatigued to perform an 11th repetition. Quickly set down the 30-pound dumbbells, pick up 25-pound dumbbells, and do as many additional repetitions as possible. By immediately performing a few lower resistance biceps curls, you can force your muscles to a deeper level of fatigue and stimulate a better training response.

Because this is a difficult training technique, it should not be used every workout. After performing breakdown repetitions, your muscles may require more recovery time to build higher strength levels prior to your next strength workout.

If you train with a partner, you may achieve a similar training effect by doing "assisted repetitions." In this case, your partner assists you with a few additional repetitions after your fatigue point.

As in the previous example, you may complete 10 biceps curls with 30-pound dumbbells, but find your biceps muscles are too fatigued to perform another repetition. Then your partner places his or her hands on the dumbbells and helps you lift them an 11th time. Your partner gives just enough assistance to help you accomplish the lifting movement, but allows you to do the lowering movement on your own. This is possible because muscles can lower more weight than they can lift.

When done properly, two to four assisted repetitions produce a high level of muscle fatigue and provide a greater strengthening stimulus. As with breakdown repetitions, you should not perform assisted repetitions too frequently. Due to the increased training demands, you may require more recovery time to build higher strength levels prior to your next workout.

# INTERMEDIATE
# STRENGTH TRAINING PROGRAM

| Monday | Sets | Repetitions |
|---|---|---|
| Leg Extension (M) | 1 | 8-12 with 2-4 breakdowns |
| Leg Curl (M) | 1 | 8-12 with 2-4 breakdowns |
| Barbell Bench Press (F) | 2-3 | 8-12 |
| One-Arm Dumbbell Row (F) | 2-3 | 8-12 |
| Dumbbell Lateral Raise (F) | 2-3 | 8-12 |
| Dumbbell Arm Curl (F) | 1 | 8-12 with 2-4 assisted repetitions |
| Dumbbell Triceps Kickback (F) | 1 | 8-12 with 2-4 assisted repetitions |
| Trunk Curl (F) | 1-3 | 8-12 |

| Wednesday | Sets | Repetitions |
|---|---|---|
| Leg Extension (M) | 2-3 | 8-12 |
| Leg Curl (M) | 2-3 | 8-12 |
| Barbell Incline Press (F) | 1-2 | 8-12 immediately followed by |
| Chest Press (M) | 1-2 | 8-12 |
| Lat Pulldown (M) | 1 | 8-12 with 2-4 breakdowns |
| Dumbbell Lateral Raise (F) | 1 | 8-12 immediately followed by |
| Shoulder Press (M) | 1 | 8-12 |
| Dumbbell Arm Curl (F) | 1-2 | 8-12 |
| Dumbbell Triceps Kickback (F) | 1-2 | 8-12 |
| Trunk Curl (F) | 1-3 | 8-12 |

| Friday | Sets | Repetitions |
|---|---|---|
| Barbell Squat (F) | 2-3 | 8-12 |
| Barbell Bench Press (F) | 2-3 | 8-12 |
| Lat Pulldown (M) | 2-3 | 8-12 |
| Shoulder Press (M) | 2-3 | 8-12 |
| Arm Curl (M) | 2-3 | 8-12 |
| Triceps Extension (M) | 2-3 | 8-12 |
| Trunk Curl (F) | 2-3 | 8-12 |

If you are not limited to a specific training time, you may consider adding more exercises to your workout program. For example, if you experience a plateau in your biceps muscles, you may stimulate further progress with an additional biceps exercise. One option is to follow dumbbell arm curls with chin-ups. Both exercises target the biceps muscles, but use different movement patterns and require different muscle fiber activation. Just remember that more biceps work may require more recovery time between successive training sessions to build higher levels of strength.

Consider the example of an intermediate strength training program that incorporates several of the suggested methods for increasing your training effort. Note that in the workouts in chapters 12 and 13, (M) refers to machine exercises and (F) to free-weight exercises.

# ENDURANCE TRAINING WORKOUTS

Endurance training, also known as aerobic activity, enhances your cardiovascular fitness. Regular endurance exercise improves the pumping capacity of your heart and the efficiency of your circulatory system. In addition to these important health benefits, endurance exercise enables you to perform more work with less effort.

As with strength exercise, an endurance training program should begin at your present state of cardiovascular fitness. Fortunately, the training guidelines for endurance exercise are broad enough to accommodate various levels of aerobic activity. Consider the following endurance training recommendations from the American College of Sports Medicine.

1. Perform endurance exercise 3 to 5 days per week.
2. Train vigorously enough to raise your heart rate to about 60-90 percent of your maximum heart rate (MHR).
3. Perform 20 to 60 minutes of continuous aerobic activity.
4. Use a large muscle exercise that is rhythmic in nature, such as walking, jogging, cycling, stepping, swimming, rowing, cross-country skiing, or aerobic dancing.

Although these standard training guidelines are applicable to most beginning exercisers, not everyone can start with 20 minutes of continuous endurance activity. Also, some types of aerobic training are more physically demanding than others. It is therefore important to individualize your exercise program as much as possible. Consider the following progressions for the initial stages of your endurance training program.

## BEGINNER PROGRAM

It is important to progress gradually in your mode of exercise, as well as in your training frequency, intensity, and duration. For example, if you are overweight or out of shape, it may be best to begin with recumbent cycling. The recumbent cycle supports both your body weight and your back as you exercise. In addition, the more horizontal body position facilitates blood circulation and places less stress on your heart.

Once you have improved your cardiovascular fitness, you may progress to upright cycling. The traditional cycle supports your body weight but permits a more vertical body position.

As you approach a moderate conditioning level, you may move to a body weight activity such as treadmill walking. Although somewhat more vigorous than body support exercise, the dominant movement pattern is horizontal.

Your next progression may be to a stepping/stair-climbing machine. These exercises use your body weight in a vertical movement pattern that is more physically demanding.

Of course, rowing and cross-country ski machines may provide more vigorous workouts because they require both upper body and lower body exercise. Once you have attained a higher level of cardiovascular fitness, a variety of aerobic activities may be advisable for avoiding boredom, reducing the risk of overuse injuries, and attaining more comprehensive conditioning benefits.

If you are a beginner, you may initially require brief bouts of endurance exercise, starting with as few as 6 minutes of light cycling. As you become more fit, you may gradually increase your training duration up to 20 minutes or more. Some individuals prefer to exercise at a lower intensity for a longer period of time. However, 20 minutes of continuous aerobic activity at an appropriate heart rate provides excellent cardiovascular benefits.

Generally speaking, an appropriate exercise heart rate for a 20-minute training session is about 70 to 80 percent of MHR.

You should begin each cycling session at a lower pedal resistance and gradually increase your training level. Likewise, you should finish each cycling session by gradually decreasing the pedal resistance for a cool-down effect.

As you become more fit, you may vary your cycling program by performing interval training; that is, intersperse a few higher effort intervals with lower effort intervals. Or select a few of the training programs outlined in chapter 7.

You should begin each stepping session with a lower intensity climbing effort and gradually increase to your training level. Likewise, you should finish each stepping session by gradually decreasing the exercise effort for a cool-down effect.

As you become more fit, you may vary your stepping program by performing interval training; that is, intersperse a few higher effort intervals with lower effort intervals. Or incorporate some of the programs outlined in chapter 8.

## BEGINNER STATIONARY CYCLE PROGRAM

|         | Exertion Level | Duration |
|---------|----------------|----------|
| Week 1: | Easy | 6-12 minutes |
| Week 2: | Easy | 10-16 minutes |
| Week 3: | Moderate | 14-20 minutes |
| Week 4: | Moderate | 18-24 minutes |
| Week 5: | Moderate | 22-28 minutes |
| Week 6: | Slightly higher or | 20 minutes |
|         | slightly lower | 30 minutes |
| Week 7: | Interval training | Alternate 4 minutes at moderate exertion with 2 minutes at higher exertion for about 24 minutes |

You should begin each walking session at a slower pace and gradually increase your training level. Likewise, you should finish each walking session by gradually decreasing your pace for a cool-down effect. As you become more fit, you may vary your walking program by performing interval training; that is, try to intersperse a few higher effort intervals (faster speed or higher incline) with lower effort intervals. Chapter 9 offers additional programs to add variety to your workouts.

You should begin each skiing session at a slower pace and gradually increase your training level. Likewise, you should finish each skiing session by gradually decreasing your pace for a cool-down effect. As you become more fit, you may vary your skiing program by performing interval training; that is, try to intersperse a few higher effort intervals with lower effort intervals. Review chapter 10 for more suggestions on skiing workouts.

## BEGINNER STAIR CLIMBER PROGRAM

| | Exertion Level | Duration |
|---|---|---|
| Week 1: | Easy | 6-12 minutes |
| Week 2: | Easy | 10-16 minutes |
| Week 3: | Moderate | 14-20 minutes |
| Week 4: | Moderate | 18-24 minutes |
| Week 5: | Moderate | 22-28 minutes |
| Week 6: | Slightly higher or | 20 minutes |
| | slightly lower | 30 minutes |
| Week 7: | Interval training | Alternate 4 minutes at moderate exertion with 2 minutes at higher exertion for 24 minutes |

## BEGINNER TREADMILL PROGRAM

| | Exertion Level | Duration |
|---|---|---|
| Week 1: | Easy | 6-12 minutes |
| Week 2: | Easy | 10-16 minutes |
| Week 3: | Moderate | 14-20 minutes |
| Week 4: | Moderate | 18-24 minutes |
| Week 5: | Moderate | 22-28 minutes |
| Week 6: | Slightly higher or | 20 minutes |
| | slightly lower | 30 minutes |
| Week 7: | Add interval training | 3 minutes at moderate exertion with 3 minutes at higher exertion for 24 minutes |

---

### BEGINNER CROSS-COUNTRY SKI MACHINE PROGRAM

|  | Exertion Level | Duration |
|---|---|---|
| Week 1: | Easy | 6-12 minutes |
| Week 2: | Easy | 10-16 minutes |
| Week 3: | Moderate | 14-20 minutes |
| Week 4: | Moderate | 18-24 minutes |
| Week 5: | Moderate | 22-28 minutes |
| Week 6: | Slightly higher or | 20 minutes |
|  | slightly lower | 30 minutes |
| Week 7: | Add interval training | Alternate 3 minutes at moderate exertion with 3 minutes at higher exertion for 24 minutes |

## INTERMEDIATE PROGRAM

As you progress to intermediate status as an endurance exerciser, you may choose to perform interval training on a regular and systematic basis. You may want to use a more subjective or a more objective means for determining your exercise effort during your interval training sessions.

With the subjective method you simply estimate how hard you are exercising compared to an all-out (100 percent) effort. For example, an easy workout segment might correspond to a 60 percent exercise effort, a moderate workout segment might correspond to a 70 percent exercise effort, and a hard workout segment might correspond to an 80 percent exercise effort.

The objective method requires checking your exercise heart rate, accomplished by periodically taking your pulse or wearing a commercial heart rate monitor. During interval training, your heart rate may be about 65 percent of maximum during the easy segments, and about 80 percent of maximum during the hard segments.

A standard way of estimating your maximum heart rate is to subtract your age from 220. For example, if your age is 40, your maximum heart rate is approximately 180 beats per minute. Therefore, during the easy intervals your exercise effort may elevate your heart rate to about 120 beats per minute (65 percent of 180). During the hard intervals your exercise effort may elevate your heart rate to about 145 beats per minute (80 percent of 180).

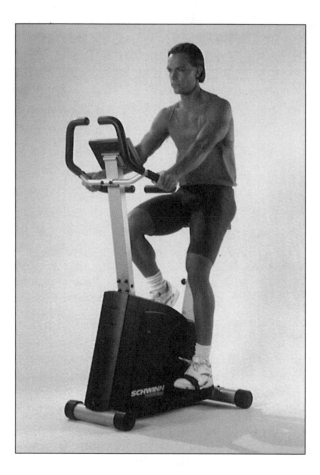

Once you have established your training heart rate zone for interval exercise, you can design an appropriate training program to further develop your cardiovascular fitness. Generally speaking, the length of your workout session will remain about the same; however, by alternately performing higher effort and lower effort exercise intervals, you should experience a better training stimulus. The duration of each interval depends largely upon your physical condition.

For example, if you are in good cardiovascular shape, you can begin with a 3-minute light warm-up. You may then perform a 2-minute hard interval followed by a 2-minute easy interval, and repeat this procedure for about 20 minutes. You may then conclude your workout with a 3-minute cool-down.

If you are in very good cardiovascular shape, you may be able to handle 4-minute hard intervals interspersed with 2-minute easy intervals. If you are in excellent cardiovascular shape, you may be able to sustain 6-minute hard intervals at 80 percent of your MHR, alternated with 2-minute easy intervals.

The segment times for your hard and easy intervals can be determined based on your physical condition and personal preference. However, it is essential to progress gradually as you lengthen the hard intervals. It is equally important to train at the appropriate heart rates throughout your workout. Try not to exceed 80 percent of MHR during the hard intervals nor to drop below 65 percent of MHR during the easy intervals. Chapters 7 through 10 offer additional interval programs for use on various pieces of home equipment.

---

## INTERMEDIATE ENDURANCE TRAINING PROGRAM

|          | Program | Duration* |
|----------|---------|-----------|
| Week 1: | Alternate six intervals each:<br>2 minutes moderate effort<br>2 minutes higher effort | 30 minutes |
| Week 2: | Alternate five intervals each:<br>2 minutes moderate effort<br>3 minutes higher effort | 31 minutes |
| Week 3: | Alternate four intervals each:<br>2 minutes moderate effort<br>4 minutes higher effort | 30 minutes |
| Week 4: | Alternate four intervals each:<br>2 minutes moderate effort<br>5 minutes higher effort | 34 minutes |
| Week 5: | Alternate three intervals each:<br>2 minutes moderate effort<br>6 minutes higher effort | 30 minutes |

*Including warm-up and cool-down.
Note. This program is appropriate for the stationary cycle, stair climber, treadmill, and cross-country ski machine.

# CROSS-TRAINING OPTIONS

Any repetitive activity emphasizes some muscle groups and de-emphasizes other muscle groups. By performing just one type of endurance exercise, it is possible to eventually develop muscle imbalances and experience overuse injuries. To reduce the risk of overtraining and to make your exercise sessions more interesting, it is wise to consider a cross-training program.

Cross-training refers to alternating exercise activities throughout the week. For example, you might perform cycling one session and walking the next session. Some of the equipment options for cross-training include: upright exercise cycles, recumbent exercise cycles, treadmills, stepping machines, cross-country ski machines, and aerobic dance videos.

Although each of these endurance activities requires different movement patterns and muscle involvement, they all provide a similar stimulus for cardiovascular conditioning. The key is to train within your target heart rate zone for at least 20 minutes on a regular basis. The more exercises you include in your training program, the more likely you will be a lifetime fitness participant.

Consider the following example of an intermediate cross-training program that incorporates some of the recommended methods for increasing your training effort.

# WARM-UPS AND COOL-DOWNS

In addition to starting and ending your endurance exercise at a lower effort level, you should perform a general warm-up at the beginning and a general cool-down at the end of each training session. The purpose of the warm-up is to avoid an abrupt change from rest to vigorous activity. In a similar manner, the cool-down provides a smooth transition from the exercise state to the resting state. This is particularly important for facilitating blood return to the heart and avoiding cardiovascular complications.

Generally speaking, warm-ups and cool-downs are somewhat similar in nature. Both transition activities should include some mild

# INTERMEDIATE CROSS-TRAINING PROGRAM

| Monday | Exertion Level | Duration |
|---|---|---|
| Stationary cycle | 65% of MHR | 4 minutes |
| | 80% of MHR | 4 minutes |
| | 65% of MHR | 2 minutes |
| | 80% of MHR | 4 minutes |
| | 65% of MHR | 2 minutes |
| | 80% of MHR | 4 minutes |
| | 65% of MHR | 4 minutes |

| Wednesday | Exertion Level | Duration |
|---|---|---|
| Cross-country ski machine | 60% of MHR | 5 minutes |
| | 80% of MHR | 3 minutes |
| | 70% of MHR | 3 minutes |
| | 80% of MHR | 3 minutes |
| | 70% of MHR | 3 minutes |
| | 80% of MHR | 3 minutes |
| | 60% of MHR | 5 minutes |

| Friday | Exertion Level | Duration |
|---|---|---|
| Treadmill | 65% of MHR | 5 minutes |
| | 80% of MHR | 3 minutes |
| | 70% of MHR | 3 minutes |
| | 80% of MHR | 3 minutes |
| | 70% of MHR | 3 minutes |
| | 80% of MHR | 3 minutes |
| | 65% of MHR | 5 minutes |

| Saturday | Exertion Level | Duration |
|---|---|---|
| Stair climber | 65% of MHR | 4 minutes |
| | 80% of MHR | 4 minutes |
| | 65% of MHR | 2 minutes |
| | 80% of MHR | 4 minutes |
| | 65% of MHR | 2 minutes |
| | 80% of MHR | 4 minutes |
| | 65% of MHR | 4 minutes |

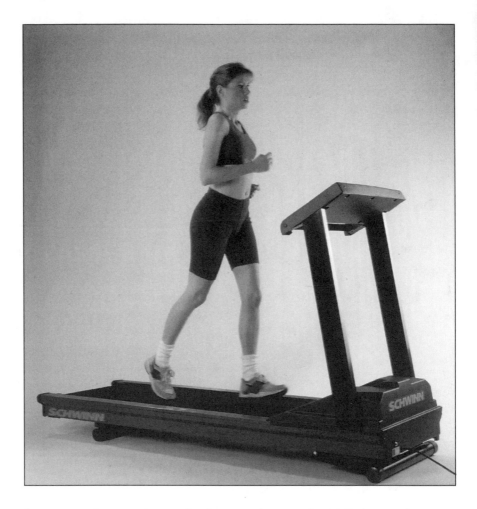

large-muscle exercise and a few gentle stretches. High-impact exercises such as jumping jacks and ballistic stretches such as windmill toe touches should be avoided.

An appropriate warm-up sequence might include a few minutes of walking, marching in place with a high knee lift, and stretches (see chapter 4). The heart rate should be increased before stretching, to avoid injuring cold muscles. An effective cool-down sequence might begin with slow walking, followed by marching in place with a low knee lift, followed by several floor-level stretching exercises. It is probably better to emphasize joint flexibility during the cool-down when the body is very warm and the muscles are more pliable.

# HOME EXERCISE PROTOCOL

Let's assume that you can schedule 1 hour, 3 days per week for your home fitness program. A safe and productive exercise protocol begins with a warm-up (about 5 minutes) and concludes with a cool-down (also about 5 minutes). The remaining 50 minutes may be equally divided between strength exercise for your muscular system and endurance exercise for your cardiovascular system. Research does not indicate any advantage for doing one activity before the other. Therefore, your personal preference should determine whether you perform strength exercise followed by endurance exercise, or vice versa. In either case, it may be beneficial to separate the two activities with a brief water break and a few stretches.

Your exercise selection and workout design are significant factors in the success of your fitness program. However, the most important consideration is training consistency. Schedule each exercise session, and keep your commitment to yourself. Of course, if you are ill or injured, cancel your workout and see an appropriate medical professional. Otherwise, exercise regularly and enjoy the health and fitness benefits of a physically active lifestyle.

# chapter 13

# Using Home Workouts for Sports

**Harvey S. Newton, MA, CSCS**

*Y*ou've learned how to put together all the components of a solid cross-training program at home. You have dedicated the necessary time to get in your workouts. And you've become familiar with dozens of exercises that can help improve your overall health fitness. But what should your program look like if you want to improve your performance in a specific sport?

This chapter offers sample workouts to enhance sport performance. For convenience, we will divide sport into three categories:

1. Endurance—mostly aerobic-based sports in which cardiovascular and muscular endurance are important (distance running or cycling, cross-country skiing)

2. Power—mostly anaerobic sports in which there are brief, powerful movements separated by rest periods (alpine skiing, tennis, basketball, volleyball, baseball, softball)

3. Skill sports—energy requirements are not great but muscular action is still needed (golf, bowling, archery)

The guidelines for developing a strength training program are identical regardless of your purpose. Too many people make the mistake of training only those muscles that are used directly in their sport. It's important to develop your strength in a balanced manner—remember, like a chain, you're only as strong as your weakest link.

As discussed in chapter 6, workouts are complete if they include four exercises that focus on one each of the following:

- Upper body pushing
- Upper body pulling
- Torso (abdominal and low back areas)
- Lower body

You can train each of these areas with more than one exercise if you wish, but remember, you're not training to become a bodybuilder. Your priority is to develop strength that will help you in your sport. You need only a few exercises to counteract any muscle imbalance caused by your sport.

The following guidelines for training apply to anyone doing resistance training. The choice of exercises in these sample workouts is often related to the sport. If your sport is not mentioned, analyze what muscles are important in improving performance, along with other supporting muscles. These programs are suitable for either males or females, young or old, depending, of course, on your ability to safely perform the exercises. Major muscle group exercises are listed for either free weights or machines, depending on which you have available. For women who want to do strength training without a particular sport in mind, general programs are offered at the end of the chapter.

# GENERAL STRENGTH TRAINING GUIDELINES

Let's say cycling is your favorite athletic activity. Initially, it looks as though the only weight training needed would be related to the leg muscles. Cyclists already have better than average leg strength. Is there a need to improve leg strength? You bet, because it will help on the hills, while sprinting, during time trials, or on a century ride. Is there a reason to address abdominal, low back, and upper body strength also? Certainly, as these areas not only help balance the total muscular picture, but added strength in these areas can actually improve performance.

An important consideration is your experience with strength training. The sample programs in this chapter are divided into two categories: beginner and advanced. If you have never performed strength training exercises, or if it has been some time since your last workout, follow the beginner programs. If you strength train regularly, you can follow the advanced programs.

If you're new to strength training, plan to just do one set of moderate repetitions (10-15) in several exercises during the first week or two. Use this time to experiment with the proper technique and seek the correct resistance for your later training. Rest about 1-1/2 minutes after each exercise before moving to the next lift.

During your second week of lifting, perform each exercise twice (two sets). Perform the first one with a relatively light weight, then add 10 to 20 percent for the second set, which you perform after resting about 1-1/2 minutes. If the exercise requires you to be seated or lying down, get up and walk around between sets.

By your third week of strength training, you should be performing three sets of each exercise. This does not include a warm-up set done before each exercise with about 50 to 60 percent of what you expect to lift that day. For example, if you can squat 180 pounds for 10 repetitions, in your first set you would lift approximately 100 pounds for 10 repetitions. Then progress to about 135 pounds for 10 repetitions, followed by about 160 pounds, and finally, 180 pounds for the final set.

# WORKOUTS FOR POWER SPORTS

Say you want to get in shape for the upcoming ski season. It's very important for a skier to be in condition prior to hitting the slopes. As the old adage says, "You can't ski yourself into shape." Don't make the mistake of thinking you can simply do one or two warm-up runs on the first day out and then pick up where you left off last year. This is true for anyone getting in shape for any power sport.

## STRENGTH TRAINING

If you're a newcomer to strength training, you should start working several months before the season starts, just to get used to the movements in a strength workout. After a few months, you can work up to more advanced programs, but start slowly and don't overdo it!

*Note:* Because you may have any combination of resistance training equipment in your home gym, the following examples of weekly workouts list a movement that can be done with free weights (denoted by F) or a comparable lift that can be performed on a machine (denoted by M). Refer to chapters 5 and 6 for proper exercise techniques and safety considerations.

What about the experienced athlete who has worked out with weights before? We're talking about people who have at least one season of *lifting* under their belt. The experienced lifter can perform

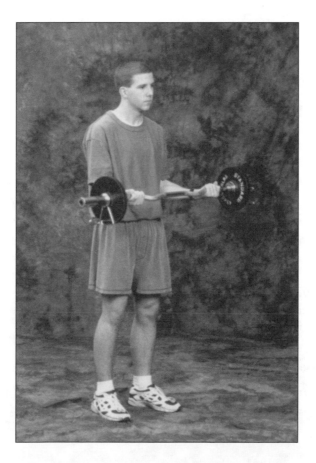

## BEGINNER STRENGTH TRAINING PROGRAM— POWER SPORTS

| Monday | Sets | Repetitions |
|---|---|---|
| Squat (F) or Leg Extension (M) | 1-3 | 10-12 |
| Bench Press (F) or Pec Deck Fly (M) | 1-3 | 10-12 |
| Bent-Over Row (F) or Low Rowing (M) | 1-3 | 10-12 |
| Trunk Curl (F) or Abdominal Crunches (M) | 1-3 | 15-20 |
| **Wednesday** | | |
| Squat (F) or Leg Extension (M) | 1-3 | 10-12 |
| Incline Bench Press (F) or Chest Press (M) | 1-3 | 10-12 |
| One-Arm Dumbbell Row (F) or Lat Pulldown (M) | 1-3 | 10-12 |
| Trunk Curl (F) or Abdominal Crunches (M) | 1-3 | 15-20 |
| Back Extension (F) | 1-3 | 12-15 |
| **Friday** | | |
| Squat (F) or Leg Extension (M) | 1-3 | 10-12 |
| Bench Press (F) or (M) | 1-3 | 10-12 |
| Upright Row (F) or Lat Pulldown (M) | 1-3 | 10-12 |
| Trunk Curl (F) or Abdominal Crunches (M) | 1-3 | 15-20 |
| Back Extension (F) | 1-3 | 12-15 |

more exercises per body part. This could include use of single-joint movements after the multiple-joint exercise has been performed. The single-joint lifts (Arm Curl, Triceps Press, etc.) tend to concentrate on a particular muscle rather than using several muscles together. The number of sets can be increased slightly. Some lifts should be performed with heavier weights and lower repetitions (6-8) to create more strength. Movements may be performed more quickly to improve power (speed, strength).

## CARDIOVASCULAR TRAINING

You will need a good cardiovascular base in order to tackle a new skiing season. While strength training will have a tremendous effect

# EXPERIENCED STRENGTH TRAINING PROGRAM— POWER SPORTS

| Monday | Sets | Repetitions |
|---|---|---|
| Squat (F) or Leg Extension (M) | 3-4 | 8-10 |
| Lunge (F) | 3 | 10 |
| Shoulder Press (behind the neck) (F) or Chest Press (M) | 3-4 | 8-10 |
| Bent-Over Row (F) or Low Rowing (M) | 3-4 | 8-10 |
| Trunk Curl (F) or Abdominal Crunches (M) | 3 | 12-15 |

| Wednesday | | |
|---|---|---|
| Good Morning (F) or Low Rowing (M) | 3-4 | 8-10 |
| Upright Row (F) or Lat Pulldown (M) | 3-4 | 8-10 |
| Arm Curl (F) or (M) | 3 | 10 |
| Triceps Press (F) or Triceps Pushdown (M) | 3 | 10 |
| Trunk Curl (F) or Abdominal Crunches (M) | 3 | 12-15 |

| Friday | | |
|---|---|---|
| Squat (F) or Leg Press (M) | 3-4 | 8-10 |
| Lunge (F) | 3 | 10 |
| Shoulder Press (F) or (M) | 3-4 | 8-10 |
| One-Arm Dumbbell Row (F) or Low Rowing (M) | 3-4 | 8-10 |
| Trunk Curl (F) or Abdominal Crunches (M) | 3 | 12-15 |

on your ability to carve better turns in skiing and aid your speed down the hill, endurance training will also allow you to ski longer and stronger, especially during those last few hours on the hill.

On your weight training days, try to spend 30 to 40 minutes at 70 to 80 percent of your MHR on a piece of aerobic equipment that will stress muscles similar to those used in your sport. On days you do not lift weights, do 5- to 10-minute intervals at 80 to 90 percent of your MHR. Consider such programs as the high-intensity song workouts on a stepper or skier, or a hill workout on your stationary bike or treadmill. Again, since many power sports also require some skill training, leave some time for practicing your turns.

# WORKOUTS FOR ENDURANCE SPORTS

The very nature of endurance sports such as cycling or running targets specific muscles in the legs while ignoring the upper body. This uneven development can lead to problems, both in efficiency of movement and in muscle imbalance. One of the primary reasons for a cyclist or runner to work out is to help avoid injuries.

## STRENGTH TRAINING

Cyclists or runners can make big improvements in the amount of power going to the pedals or the road by improving strength in the upper body and torso. Emphasis on lower body strength is important, but it is equally important to increase arm, shoulder, back, and abdominal strength.

Many endurance athletes are concerned about gaining body weight through resistance training. They think that supplemental strength training will add too much muscular bulk, which will be a hindrance in climbing hills or covering long distances. The amount of resistance

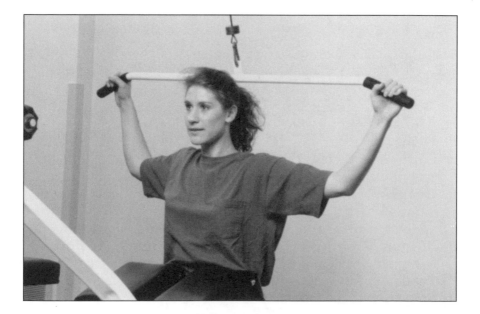

# BEGINNER STRENGTH TRAINING PROGRAM— ENDURANCE SPORTS

| Monday | Sets | Repetitions |
|---|---|---|
| Squat (F) or Leg Extension (M) | 1-3 | 10-12 |
| Shoulder Press (F) or (M) | 1-3 | 10-12 |
| Upright Row (F) | 1-3 | 10-12 |
| Trunk Curl (F) or Abdominal Crunches (M) | 1-3 | 15-20 |
| Back Extension (F) or Low Rowing (M) | 1-3 | 12-15 |

| Wednesday | | |
|---|---|---|
| Shoulder Press (with dumbbells) (F) or Chest Press (M) | 1-3 | 10-12 |
| One-Arm Dumbbell Row (F) or Lat Pulldown (M) | 1-3 | 10-12 |
| Heel Raise (F) or (M) | 1-3 | 15-20 |
| Trunk Curl (F) or Abdominal Crunches (M) | 1-3 | 15-20 |
| Back Extension (F) | 1-3 | 12-15 |

| Friday | | |
|---|---|---|
| Squat (F) or Leg Extension (M) | 1-3 | 10-12 |
| Triceps Press (F) or Triceps Pushdown (M) | 1-3 | 10-12 |
| Forward Raise (F) or (M) | 1-3 | 10-12 |
| Upright Row (F) or Lat Pulldown (M) | 1-3 | 10-12 |
| Trunk Curl (F) or Abdominal Crunches (M) | 1-3 | 15-20 |
| Back Extension (F) | 1-3 | 12-15 |

training offered in this chapter will not increase body weight, nor will it develop large, bulky muscles. Such development is a matter of specialized training, genetics, and an extreme diet plan, as used by bodybuilders.

The experienced endurance athlete will receive enough strength training for the upper body and trunk by performing one exercise per body group. However, additional work should be performed for the dominant muscle group (i.e., legs for cyclists or runners). This work should be separated 8 to 24 hours from any high-intensity or long-duration endurance work such as interval training.

## EXPERIENCED STRENGTH TRAINING PROGRAM— ENDURANCE SPORTS

| Monday | Sets | Repetitions |
|---|---|---|
| Squat (F) or Leg Extension (M) | 3-4 | 8-10 |
| Good Morning (F) or Low Rowing (M) | 3 | 10 |
| Shoulder Press (behind the neck) (F) or Chest Press (M) | 3-4 | 8-10 |
| One-Arm Dumbbell Row (F) or Upright Rowing (M) | 3-4 | 8-10 |
| Heel Raise (F) or (M) | 3 | 15 |
| Trunk Curl (F) or Abdominal Crunches (M) | 3 | 12-15 |

| Wednesday | | |
|---|---|---|
| Lunge (F) or Leg Extension (M) | 3-4 | 8-10 |
| Leg Curl (M) | 3-4 | 10-12 |
| Bent-Over Row (F) or Lat Pulldown (M) | 3-4 | 8-10 |
| Arm Curl (F) or (M) | 3 | 10 |
| Triceps Kickback (F) or Triceps Pushdown (M) | 3 | 10 |
| Heel Raise (F) or (M) | 3 | 15 |
| Trunk Curl (F) or Abdominal Crunches (M) | 3 | 12-15 |

| Friday | | |
|---|---|---|
| Squat (F) or Leg Extension (M) | 3-4 | 8-10 |
| Lunge (F) | 3 | 10 |
| Shoulder Press (F) or (M) | 3-4 | 8-10 |
| Stiff-Leg Dead Lift (F) or Low Rowing (M) | 3-4 | 8-10 |
| Heel Raise (F) or (M) | 3 | 15 |
| Trunk Curl (F) or Abdominal Crunches (M) | 3 | 12-15 |

## CARDIOVASCULAR TRAINING

To build cardiovascular, or aerobic, endurance (70 to 80 percent of MHR), you should exercise for extended periods of time. In addition to aerobic endurance training, you should train at intensities higher than 80 percent of MHR one or two days per week to develop your anaerobic endurance.

On the days you do resistance training, consider spending 30 to 40 minutes training on your treadmill, stationary bicycle, stepper, or skier. Keep these sessions in the aerobic heart rate zone and leave your hardest efforts for the weights. On Tuesdays and Thursdays, work out for 30 to 40 minutes at a higher intensity on your aerobic equipment. Programs similar to hill or ladder workouts on the stationary bike or the pyramid workout on the treadmill would be appropriate for this type of training. Remember to take one or two days off per week to help with recovery.

# WORKOUTS FOR SKILL SPORTS

Golfers and bowlers may be tempted to rely on their sport skills rather than physical conditioning for success. Systematic training is embraced by most serious athletes as a way to stay ahead of the competition. Good conditioning will also help you avoid nagging injuries that might interfere with your technique.

## STRENGTH TRAINING

Can skill sport athletes such as a golfers or bowlers improve their performance by getting stronger? You bet they can! In a recent study of average golfers, subjects showed a 5-mph increase in the force used to drive a golf ball after implementing a weight training program. Again, two key benefits of strength training are improved muscular balance and increased flexibility. Both can have a very positive effect on one's game.

After several months of beginning workouts, a golfer or bowler may choose to include more exercises in his or her program. Beginner and experienced workouts for skill sports are on pp. 230 and 231, respectively.

## CARDIOVASCULAR TRAINING

Increasing your cardiovascular endurance will have a significant impact on how you feel after eighteen holes of golf or several hours of bowling. Not only will including several days of cardiovascular training into your program improve your overall health and help to

## BEGINNER STRENGTH TRAINING PROGRAM— SKILL SPORTS

| Monday | Sets | Repetitions |
|---|---|---|
| Lunge (F) or Leg Extension (M) | 1-3 | 10-12 |
| Lateral Raise (F) or (M) | 3 | 10-12 |
| Arm Curl (F) or (M) | 1-3 | 10-12 |
| Bent-Over Row (F) or Lat Pulldown (M) | 1-3 | 10-12 |
| Trunk Curl (F) or Abdominal Crunches (M) | 1-3 | 15-20 |

| Wednesday | | |
|---|---|---|
| Squat (F) or Leg Extension (M) | 1-3 | 10-12 |
| Incline Bench Press (F) or Chest Press (M) | 1-3 | 10-12 |
| One-Arm Dumbbell Row (F) or Upright Rowing (M) | 1-3 | 10-12 |
| Trunk Curl (F) or Abdominal Crunches (M) | 1-3 | 15-20 |
| Back Extension (F) | 1-3 | 12-15 |

| Friday | | |
|---|---|---|
| Lunge (F) or Leg Curl (M) | 1-3 | 10-12 |
| Forward Raise (F) or (M) | 1-3 | 10-12 |
| Upright Row (F) or Lat Pulldown (M) | 1-3 | 10-12 |
| Trunk Curl (F) or Abdominal Crunches (M) | 1-3 | 15-20 |
| Back Extension (F) or (M) | 1-3 | 12-15 |

maintain body weight, but it also will maintain your skills while your less fit opponent's may be waning.

On days that you weight train, spend 30 to 40 minutes in the moderate (60 to 70 percent of MHR) heart rate zone or 20 to 30 minutes in the aerobic training zone (70 to 80 percent of MHR) on your cardiovascular home fitness equipment. On your weight training off-days spend a little longer on your cardiovascular equipment. Occasionally throw in a harder workout such as a high/low workout on a skier or an accelerate/decelerate workout on the treadmill. Remember, time spent practicing your skill sport should still be the most important part of your program.

# EXPERIENCED STRENGTH TRAINING PROGRAM— SKILL SPORTS

| Monday | Sets | Repetitions |
|---|---|---|
| Squat (F) or Leg Extension (M) | 3-4 | 8-10 |
| Lunge (F) | 3 | 10 |
| Shoulder Press (behind the neck) (F) or Pec Deck Fly (M) | 3-4 | 8-10 |
| Arm Curl (F) or (M) | 3 | 8-9 |
| Bent-Over Row (F) or (M) | 3-4 | 8-10 |
| Trunk Curl (F) or Abdominal Crunches (M) | 3 | 12-15 |
| **Wednesday** | | |
| Good Morning (F) or Low Rowing (M) | 3-4 | 8-10 |
| Upright Row (F) or Lat Pulldown (M) | 3-4 | 8-10 |
| Arm Curl (F) or (M) | 3 | 10 |
| Triceps Press (F) or Triceps Pushdown (M) | 3 | 10 |
| Trunk Curl (F) or Abdominal Crunches (M) | 3 | 12-15 |
| **Friday** | | |
| Squat (F) or Leg Press (M) | 3-4 | 8-10 |
| Lunge (F) | 3 | 10 |
| Shoulder Press (F) or (M) | 3-4 | 8-10 |
| Lateral Raise (F) or (M) | 3 | 10 |
| One-Arm Dumbbell Row (F) or Lat Pulldown (M) | 3-4 | 8-10 |
| Trunk Curl (F) or Abdominal Crunches (M) | 3 | 12-15 |

# STRENGTH TRAINING WORKOUTS FOR WOMEN

For the most part, women can train in an identical manner to men. Most women will have slightly different goals in mind than do men. Women engaged in strength training frequently want to change their overall body shape, but they are not interested in developing massive muscles. Hypertrophy, or muscular growth, is largely determined by available testosterone, genetics, diet, and training regimen. The type of training described in this section is not going to produce large muscles, but it will help improve total fitness.

Women need to pay particular attention to their upper body strength, which tends to be about two-thirds that of men. Lower body strength is actually about equal to men's, if we correct for differences in body composition. Generally speaking, women need not be concerned with the development of large, bulky muscles. They can benefit from greatly increasing their strength and changing body outline.

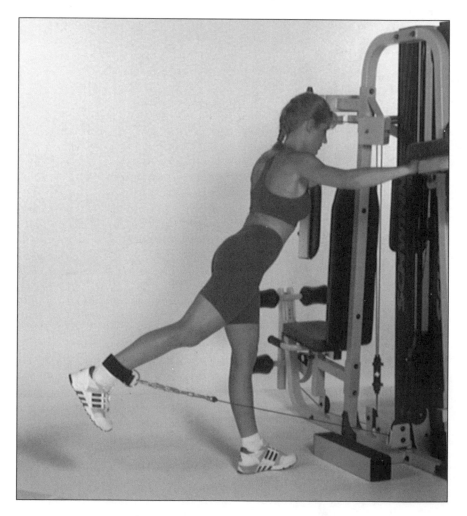

## BEGINNER STRENGTH TRAINING PROGRAM FOR WOMEN

| Monday | Sets | Repetitions |
|---|---|---|
| Lunge (F) | 1-3 | 12-15 |
| Lat Pulldown (M) | 1-3 | 12-15 |
| Chest Press (M) | 1-3 | 12-15 |
| Trunk Curl (F) or Abdominal Crunches (M) | 1-3 | 15-25 |
| Back Extension (F) | 1-3 | 12-15 |
| **Wednesday** | | |
| Leg Extension (M) | 1-3 | 12-15 |
| Leg Curl (M) | 1-3 | 12-15 |
| Low Rowing (M) | 1-3 | 12-15 |
| Shoulder Press (seated) (M) | 1-3 | 12-15 |
| Trunk Curl (F) or Abdominal Crunches (M) | 1-3 | 15-25 |
| **Friday** | | |
| Lunge (F) | 1-3 | 12-15 |
| Leg Extension (M) | 1-3 | 12-15 |
| Chest Press (M) | 1-3 | 12 |
| Lat Pulldown (M) | 1-3 | 12-15 |
| Back Extension (F) | 1-3 | 12 |
| Trunk Curl (F) or Abdominal Crunches (M) | 1-3 | 15-25 |

Pregnant women should always consult their doctor for advice on fitness training during pregnancy. It is important to consider training *before* becoming pregnant, as being an expectant mother is not the optimal time to start a fitness program.

# FINAL SET

You'll notice that no two workouts within a week are identical. Feel free to use the same workout over and over again if you wish, but adding variety to the workout serves two purposes: (a) it stimulates

# EXPERIENCED STRENGTH TRAINING PROGRAM FOR WOMEN

| Monday | Sets | Repetitions |
|---|---|---|
| Lunge (F) or Leg Extension (M) | 3-4 | 10-12 |
| Bent-Over Row (F) or Lat Pulldown (M) | 3-4 | 10-12 |
| Bench Press (F) or Pec Deck Fly (M) | 3-4 | 10-12 |
| Trunk Curl (F) or Abdominal Crunches (M) | 5 | 12 |
| Good Morning (F) or Low Rowing (M) | 4 | 10-12 |
| **Wednesday** | | |
| Squat (F) or Leg Extension (M) | 5 | 10 |
| Leg Curl (M) | 3 | 12 |
| Upright Row (F) or Low Rowing (M) | 4 | 10-12 |
| Lateral Raise (F) or Shoulder Press (seated) (M) | 3 | 12 |
| Trunk Curl (F) or Abdominal Crunches (M) | 4 | 15 |
| **Friday** | | |
| Lunge (F) or Leg Press (M) | 3 | 12 |
| Leg Extension (M) | 3 | 12 |
| Incline Bench Press (F) or Chest Press (M) | 4 | 10 |
| Upright Row (F) or Lat Pulldown (M) | 4 | 10-12 |
| Back Extension (F) or Low Rowing (M) | 3 | 12 |
| Trunk Curl (F) or Abdominal Crunches (M) | 4-3 | 10-12 |

the same muscle from a different angle, thus promoting progress; and (b) it makes your workouts a lot more interesting! Of course, if you want to make progress in a particular lift, such as the bench press, doing this exercise during all three weekly workouts will bring about improvement more quickly.

On the other hand, if you simply want to be sure you do an upper body pushing exercise on each of your workout days, go ahead and use a different one each workout. The muscles involved will be nearly identical and you won't have to worry about workout boredom.

Strength training has many advantages. You'll enjoy seeing positive changes in your body, and you'll enjoy making progress in individual exercises. Along the way, your strength training should help you improve in your chosen sport. But don't forget one other important consideration—it's fun!

# chapter 14

# Selecting Equipment for Your Home

## Edmund R. Burke, PhD

*A*s the previous chapters have shown, the reasons for setting up a home fitness center and the benefits that accrue are numerous, but before you go running off to your local fitness equipment store, it's important to be as well informed as possible. There is no shortage of companies manufacturing and marketing exercise equipment. Unfortunately, much of the information they provide is not helpful and is too technical; it's easy to wind up feeling so confused or intimidated that you postpone the decision to set up a home fitness center.

Not to worry! Developing your own fitness center may not necessarily be a quick process, but it's actually a simple one. It's just a matter of answering some basic questions, knowing what to look for in the type of equipment you want, and test driving the equipment before you buy it.

There is no one definition of what constitutes a home fitness center. It can be as simple and efficient as a few dumbbells, a stationary bike, and an exercise mat in the corner of your basement. Or it can be an elaborate 1,500-square-foot room with large windows, every imaginable piece of aerobic equipment, a large multistation machine, and a large video/stereo system. It can also fall anywhere between the two. Your needs and your budget will determine the scope, size, and sophistication of your home gym.

If you are 35 or older, have high blood pressure or other risk factors for coronary heart disease, or back problems or other musculoskeletal disorders, see your doctor before embarking on any exercise program. He or she may have some suggestions on what equipment to purchase or may steer you away from equipment that may not be right for you.

Start slowly and with modest goals when using new equipment, and make sure you know how to use it. Each year thousands of individuals are injured while using exercise equipment. In particular, don't let children play with equipment unsupervised.

Find a way to make exercise enjoyable. One advantage to home workouts is that you can read, watch television, or listen to music while you're at it.

# GETTING THE MOST FOR YOUR MONEY

Once you've decided that exercising at home is the way to go, you won't miss dragging yourself off to a crowded club—only to wait in line for a piece of equipment or be bombarded with loud music you don't even like. But don't make the mistake of thinking you'll be satisfied with just a stationary bike and a couple of dumbbells in the corner of your dark basement. Before you go out and start purchasing equipment, you'll need a simple plan of action based on your budget and the space you have available.

Most home gyms fall into three categories, which we'll call the Minimalist, the Sensible Setup, and the King of Home Gyms. Each has a different price tag and equipment parameters (see Table 14.1). How much money you can spend and how many square feet you can spare will determine the nature of your home training environment.

The Minimalist gym requires less than 20 square feet of floor space and need not be dedicated exclusively to exercise. It may be in a corner of the basement or utility room, or in the garage if your living space is at a premium. It has a minimum of equipment, some of which can be easily stored in the closet. The estimated cost is between $500 and $3,500.

The Sensible Setup requires about 60 to 100 square feet, most of which is devoted to the equipment. Each piece of equipment is

| Table 14.1    Home Gym Equipment Parameters |

| Type of gym | Cardiovascular equipment (one or more) | Weight equipment (one or more) |
| --- | --- | --- |
| Minimalist | Stair climber<br>Stationary bike<br>Cross-country ski machine | Dumbbells (adjustable)<br>Barbells (adjustable)<br>Padded bench<br>Exercise mat<br>Small multistation gym<br>Miscellaneous accessories (belts, gloves) |
| Sensible Setup | Stationary bike<br>Treadmill<br>Stair climber<br>Cross-country ski machine<br>Heart rate monitor | Dumbbells (nonadjustable) and dumbbell rack<br>Barbell set (minimal amount of weight)<br>Adjustable padded bench<br>Exercise mat<br>Multistation gym |
| King of Home Gyms | Electronic stationary bike<br>Stair climber<br>Cross-country ski machine<br>Treadmill<br>Heart rate monitor | Dumbbells and dumbbell rack<br>Adjustable padded bench<br>Squat or power rack<br>Olympic bars and weights<br>Miscellaneous special-function resistance machines<br>Miscellaneous accessories (belts, gloves) |

carefully chosen for maximum efficiency and benefit at reasonable cost. The estimated cost of this setup is between $2,000 and $7,000.

The King of Home Gyms requires an entire room of its own strictly for equipment. The minimum space required is 130 to 150 square feet, roughly the size of a small bedroom. Your gym can get as big as your house—and budget—will allow; many first-class home gyms range from 400 to 1,500 square feet. The estimated cost is between $5,000 and $25,000.

## ENVIRONMENTAL CONCERNS

You'll exercise longer and more productively if you're in a comfortable environment. Make sure you have enough room—you don't

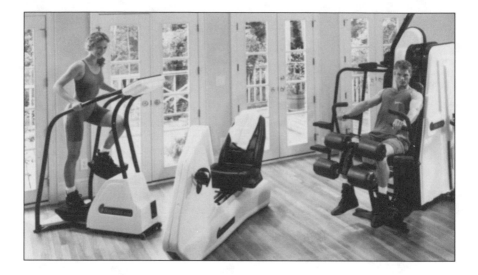

want to feel cramped or constrained while exercising. Restrict the use of barbells or dumbbells to a designated area.

Proper cooling and fluid replacement are crucial to an efficient exercise session on aerobic machines. You have to dress not only for comfort but to avoid overheating. Three-quarters of the energy your body is producing is converted to heat rather than energy to help your muscles pedal, ski, step, or run. While out on the road, you are able to dissipate heat rather well because of the wind cooling your body. This is not possible indoors, so dressing in lightweight, breathable clothing is essential. Try setting up your equipment in a room with air conditioning, or set up a fan (the larger the better) to blow air across your upper body.

In addition, make sure you drink plenty of fluids during your training sessions, ingesting one to one and a half bottles per hour depending on the intensity of effort and your sweating rate. Keeping you body cool and rehydrated while training indoors will enable you to train with greater efficiency and concentration.

Finally, good lighting will energize your workouts, so train in a room that is well lighted, preferably one with windows.

## SHOPPING SMART CHECKLIST

Before you buy equipment, always try it out to make sure it is comfortable, easy to use, and fits your body. Stores generally have floor models that you can test. Compare different models, trying them out for a few minutes each. Or check them out at a health club or at a friend's home gym. This is important for tall, short, or very heavy people who may not fit onto some machines. Check display models to see how they have stood up to use.

✓ What are my fitness goals? If they're aerobic fitness and weight loss, then a bicycle or stairclimber, treadmill, or ski machine are your best bet. If you're looking for strength and muscular development, free weights or a multistation machine are what you want.

✓ What sports interest me? Running? Weight lifting? Skiing?

✓ Buy equipment that you will use. Try out equipment in a commercial gym for several weeks before buying. Chances are, what you like in the gym you'll also like at home.

✓ Obtain product information from various manufacturers. Organize the information by category and type. Evaluate the various companies in terms of service record, scientific merit of claims, amenities offered, and price.

✓ Shop around. Prices vary so widely, and list prices are not what equipment usually sells for in retail outlets. Also, be sure to inquire about discounts and upcoming sales.

✓ Measure your available fitness space carefully. Make sure the equipment you intend to purchase will fit through the doors of your home. Will you be able to move around the equipment comfortably, once it is set up in the room? When you stand on a stair stepper, will your head go through the ceiling? Create a floor plan (equipment layout). Know what type of power supply is needed to run each piece of equipment.

✓ Come to the store prepared to use the equipment you're interested in for several minutes. Don't just take the salesperson's word for it. Make sure that it is adjustable (without sacrificing or compromising performance). Is it state of the art in terms of both design and safety, and is it user friendly for everyone in your family?

✓ It's also important to know what injuries and medical conditions might rule out your using certain types of home exercise equipment.

✓ Inquire into the warranty service. If it comes to a choice between two similar machines, choose the one with the better warranty service. Ask whether the dealership is responsible for warranty service, what they charge for service, and the most important question of all—whether they provide in-home service.

✓ Buy the best equipment you can afford. This doesn't necessarily mean the most expensive. Look for quality equipment, manufactured by a company with a well-known name and a reputation for standing behind its products. The old adage, "You get what you pay for," applies to everything you buy, including home fitness equipment.

✓ Think ahead. Keep in mind all equipment purchases you intend to make in the future: strength, aerobic, and flexibility. If you are buying a weight stack machine, think about what you should purchase next—dumbbells, a mat for stretching, a stair stepper.

✓ Consider buying quality used equipment. Work only with a reputable dealer who will give you a warranty and stand behind the product if service is needed. Ask for a trial period, and be sure you receive all instruction manuals with the unit.

✓ When buying used equipment (or new equipment for that matter), it may be prudent to stick with proven brand names. The problem isn't that lesser known brands aren't good machines, but that many manufacturers have already gone out of business, so 2 years down the line, when your treadmill needs servicing, you won't be able to find the parts.

✓ Purchase the equipment—with confidence.

# OTHER FITNESS EQUIPMENT

In addition to the treadmills, stair climbers, cross-country ski machines, and strength training equipment covered above, there is a mind-boggling array of other products that can serve as useful tools. We have selected a few that will enhance your workouts or be helpful in monitoring and maintaining your fitness levels.

## SLIDE BOARDS

Slide boards are typically two-piece units consisting of a polymer sliding sheet placed over a rubber base mat to keep the board from sliding out of position. The base mat also functions as a damper to further reduce impact forces that occur during push-off and stopping. Resistance is obtained as the thin gliding surface conforms to

## Is It Safe?

One of your primary concerns in selecting equipment should be: Is it safe for me and my family? Sensible safety features are often what separate the department store model from the fitness store model. Here's what to look for.

Bikes: All moving parts should be covered—even if there is a visible wheel, the spokes or wind fans should be enclosed and the enclosure should be kidproof. Look for a sturdy saddle, high-quality components, and a bike with a stable base.

Treadmills: Look for an emergency stop feature—a stop button or a safety belt you put around your waist that attaches to the machine. The machine will automatically shut off if the belt breaks away. The machine should also have an automatic slow starting speed of less than 2 mph. The motor and wiring should be enclosed, and front and side rails are desirable.

Stair climbers: A sturdy base and stepping mechanism—make sure the climber does not wobble when stepping under heavy loads. Automatic stop—when you stop, so should the climber. The machine should have handrails, and the mechanical parts and wiring should be enclosed.

Ski machines: Many of the best ski machines have rails with footpads that may slide off if you're an inexperienced user. They may not be the best choice if you have small children or clumsy family members.

Weight machines: Moving weight stacks should be situated so they won't catch clothing or body parts and shielded, where possible, preferably with plastic or metal. Look for machines made with parts—cables, handles, pins, pulleys, and so on—made of high-quality materials. Weight machines should allow for correct biomechanical positioning; no station on the machine should place your body in a position that increases the chance of injury. A well-built frame, sturdy construction, and strong materials are essential.

the compressible base mat. By altering the firmness of the base mat, the user can alter the resistance of the gliding surface and the effort required to move from side to side. This allows you to obtain the feel of skating on fast or slow ice or skiing on firm or soft snow. Do not use a board on carpet because most carpets are too soft to allow for proper gliding.

Slide boards come with permanent or movable bumpers at each end—usually angled at 20 to 40 degrees. Stay away from boards that have hard vertical bumpers because of the potential for ankle and knee injury upon impact.

Board length varies from 6 to 12 feet from most suppliers. Boards with movable bumpers can be lengthened for specific exercises or as your technique and strength improve. Board width is also important. To ensure having enough room to maneuver, purchase a board that is at least 30 inches wide.

A pair of shoe covers is supplied with each slide board, and a pair of clean socks can also be used. Shoe covers allow for smooth sliding, but make sure the covers and board stay clean, and polish the board periodically with inexpensive furniture polish.

In observing athletes using the slide boards at the Olympic Training Center in Colorado Springs, I find that they usually pick up the basic sliding movement very quickly. With a few practice sessions, you should be able to move laterally without hesitation.

Prices for slide boards vary from $80 to several hundred dollars, but in my experience, the less expensive portable boards are adequate for working out at home. Why not add this lateral training device to your training arsenal? A slide board allows you to do dynamic, cardiovascular training in a limited space when it is difficult to get outside.

## ROWING MACHINE

Rowing machines come in a wide variety of models and prices, ranging from low-tech versions that sell for less than $100 to the game-like Liferower for around $2,700. Piston models, which use hydraulic pistons for resistance, are inexpensive and easy to store. There are several good manufacturers of $200 to $350 models, including Pro Form and Precor. Flywheel-type machines, which use a belt rotating around a wheel for resistance, have a more realistic feel than piston models. However, they are more expensive ($650 and up) and larger than most piston models.

Look for a machine that is sturdy and stable. The frame should be long enough for you to stretch your legs out fully and comfortably. If the angle of the footrests is too severe, the bend at your ankles will be uncomfortable and may not allow a full stroke. The seat should roll easily down the track, and resistance should be smooth, with no sticking points in the stroke.

## AEROBIC STEPS

Step aerobics is an ideal low-impact conditioning program that can be done in the home with minimal equipment and space. Working to music, you step onto and off a bench in a routine that gives you an aerobic workout as it tones your buttocks and legs.

A study by San Diego State University showed that working at a rate of 120 steps per minute and pumping the arms was as physically demanding as running at 7 mph, but the impact was much lower.

Purchase a sturdy bench that is about 42 inches long by 14 inches wide, with an adjustable height and nonskid surface. Beginners should use a 4-inch step, gradually increasing the height to 8 to 12 inches. To avoid injury, your knee should not bend beyond 90 degrees as you step up. If you plan to purchase a bench for home use, take a few classes at your local health club or buy an instructional video to learn the necessary coordination and technique.

## JUMP ROPES

Jumping rope is a good low-impact exercise for the buttocks, thighs, and calves and puts minimal stress on the knees (because your feet stay close to the ground). In addition, it improves the range of motion of shoulder joints and works the upper arm and back muscles.

Make sure you purchase a quality jump rope of long-wearing rubber or polyurethane. Choose a model with swivel handles, which will make the action smoother. Proper length is very important. When standing on the center of the rope with your feet close together, the handles should reach to just below your armpits. A rope that is too long or short will make jumping difficult.

Follow the instructions that come with the rope for proper exercise technique. Although jumping looks easy, it can quickly become exhausting if not done properly. Jumping rope can be great fun by itself or combined with a circuit training program. It is also beneficial if you participate in racket sports, volleyball, or basketball because it improves your agility and coordination.

## HEART RATE MONITORS

Thanks to modern electronics, there is now a simple, accurate way to monitor your fitness levels and heart rate. Portable wireless heart monitors are available that can measure your heart rate in your daily activities with the accuracy of expensive laboratory equipment. Currently, reliable heart rate monitors employing electrocardiographic (EKG) techniques are available at modest prices. These units, which are equipped with a comfortable chest strap and rubber-covered electrodes, transmit heart rate to a wrist-worn or handlebar-mounted unit via telemetry.

In their book, *The Cooper Clinic Cardiac Rehabilitation Program*, Dr. Neil Gordon and Larry Gibbons report that heart rate monitors work

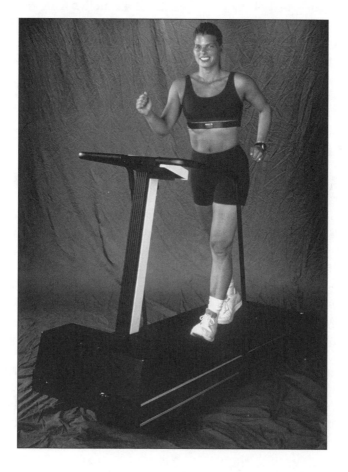

well for exercising on a stationary bicycle or walking and are generally more accurate than taking your pulse manually.

Studies published in *The Physician and Sportsmedicine* indicate excellent correlation between readings obtained by hard-wired hospital-quality EKG monitors and wireless heart rate monitors used to measure the electrical activity of the heart. These studies also pointed out the inadequacies of earlobe or fingertip photocell monitors, which can be purchased at much lower prices. These photoreflectance units measure heart rate using a photocell and light-source sensor placed on the earlobe or finger. Unfortunately, monitors of this type are sensitive to body movements and do not accurately measure the high heart rates produced while exercising.

Furthermore, the better telemetry monitors offer several additional features. Alarms can be set to correspond precisely with the upper and lower limits of your training heart rate range. When the alarm begins to beep, the digital readout shows you that it's time to increase or decrease your effort. Some units have a memory playback feature that can record your heart rate at 5-, 15-, or 60-second intervals and play it back on the wrist-worn device. The future is here with the Polar Vantage XL, which has an interface that allows you to download data from your workouts to a PC or Macintosh for analysis. Polar (800-227-1314) offers several models ranging from under $100 to several hundred dollars.

Recently, CardioSport and Sensor Dynamics introduced units that, in addition to showing you your heart rate in real time, will also display your average heart rate and calories burned while exercising. Vetta has introduced a more compact and fashionable unit that can be mounted on your handlebar as a cyclocomputer/heart rate monitor and worn after exercise as a wristwatch.

A heart rate monitor is a powerful tool for making your workouts more effective, efficient, safer, and—equally important—much more fun. Through accurate heart rate measurement, these monitors provide a physiological window into your body's response to moment-to-moment changes in your physical activity.

Using a monitor helps prevent under- or overexertion. Dr. Herman Falsetti, a cardiologist and Medical Director at Health Corp., in Irvine, California, states that the only accurate way to monitor your heart rate is with a wireless heart rate monitor while exercising outside of laboratory conditions.

Wireless monitors enable you to adhere to an exercise program based on heart rate because they give you immediate, continuous, and reliable feedback while you're exercising. They can be used comfortably while you walk, jog, cycle, or engage in any activity. Many units are water-resistant for use in swimming or water aerobics.

## READING RACKS

These convenient items attach easily to most stationary bikes, stair climbers, cross-country skiers, and other cardio machines with electronic displays. They hold books, cassette and CD players, water bottles, and so on. They can be purchased from either the manufacturer of the fitness equipment or a second-party supplier.

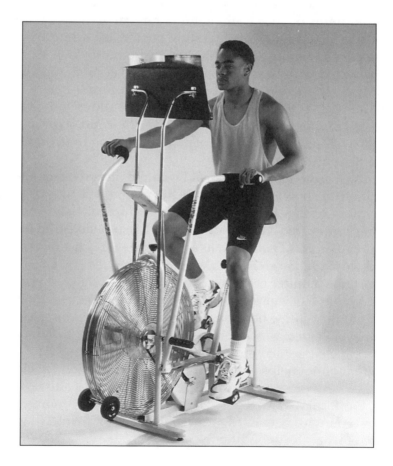

# STRETCHING CHARTS

Stretching Inc. (800-333-1307) provides a collection of more than 25 easy-to-understand charts, books, and videos on stretching, strength training, stationary cycling, and heart rate monitoring. The high-quality charts are printed on heavy paper with information clearly labeled and are laminated (optional) to protect them for many years to come. They are great for posting in your exercise room.

# SOFTWARE PROGRAMS

Like to keep track of your calories and the amount of protein in your diet, but hate trying to determine how many grams of protein, carbohydrate, and fat are in every serving of food you eat? Want to take control of your personal fitness and exercise data? If so, consider investing in fitness and nutrition software for your computer. The better programs are easy to install, easy to use, and surprisingly affordable. Once you're up to speed on them, they can be a lot of fun and provide valuable information for your training log.

No matter what type of software you plan to use, you must have the appropriate hardware. The various programs require different amounts of memory, and some programs may not be available for the type of computer you have. Be sure to read the package and sales information, as each software package has different requirements.

Comparing computer programs is a lot like comparing apples and oranges—both are fruits, high in simple sugars and low in fat, but they come in very different packages. Likewise, fitness and nutrition software programs are similar in many ways, but the way they report information and the way they present it are sometimes very different.

There are several programs on the market that can help your take control of your life. One is *Life Form* (801-221-7777), a total personal health management solution that is easy to understand and use. The product features a smart database with nutrition and calorie information, so it is quick and easy to track food intake. It also has a wide range of graphing and charting tools for exercise and medical data.

Another program that will help you maximize your health through good nutrition and exercise is *DINE Healthy* (800-688-1848). This program helps you analyze individual foods and recipes and even plans daily or weekly menus. It combines both diet and exercise analysis into one simple and easy-to-use program.

# BRINGING IT ALL HOME

Although working out indoors may not have all the elements (literally) of exercising outdoors or at the health club, training at home is a great opportunity to build all-around fitness by cross-training. But which equipment should you choose?

Figure out what appeals to you. If you like cycling, choose a stationary bike. Or if you want to tone your upper body, try a cross-country machine and a multistation weight machine. Decide which accessories will best help you monitor your fitness. A heart rate monitor? Computer software?

Another important component is the fun factor—you want to choose equipment that will motivate you to work out frequently. Whichever exercise mode(s) you choose, use the guidelines discussed in chapter 3 to ensure an adequate workout.

Being able to work out in the privacy of your home is a great feeling—you can train whenever you want, do your own thing, and create your own program to fit your needs or athletic endeavors. Setting up a quality home gym will help you stay motivated for the long haul—and it's consistency and enjoyment that are the keys to making progress and meeting your fitness goals.

# About the Authors

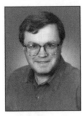

**Edmund R. Burke**, PhD, has written or edited 10 books on health, fitness, and cycling, including *Getting in Shape: Programs for Men and Women*. The executive editor of *Cycling Science* and managing editor of *Performance Conditioning for Cycling*, he has also written extensively on cycling physiology, training, nutrition, health, and fitness for *Winning Magazine, MTB Magazine, NORBA News*, and *Bicycling*. He also consults with several companies in the areas of cycling, fitness equipment design, nutritional products, and fitness programs.

Burke is certified by the National Strength and Conditioning Association (NSCA) as a strength and conditioning specialist (CSCS) and is a fellow of the American College of Sports Medicine. He is vice president of research for the NSCA and a national spokesperson for the Polar Precision Fitness Institute. An associate professor in and director of the Exercise Science Program at the University of Colorado at Colorado Springs, Burke lives in Colorado Springs with his wife, Kathleen.

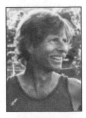

**Bob Anderson**, BS, is the author of the best-selling book, *Stretching*. He continues to give workshops on stretching to various groups across the United States and enjoys working out daily in the mountains of Colorado. Recently, he coauthored *Getting in Shape: Workout Programs for Men & Women* with Ed Burke and Bill Pearl. For information on his books, please call 1-800-333-1307.

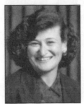

**Jacqueline R. Berning**, PhD, RD, has written several books on sports nutrition. Recently, she coauthored *Training Nutrition: The Diet and Nutrition Guide for Peak Performance* with Ed Burke. Jackie holds a master's degree in exercise science from the University of Colorado at Boulder and a doctorate in nutrition from Colorado State University. She is currently an associate professor in the Department of Biology at the University of Colorado at Colorado Springs. She is also a nutrition consultant for United States Swimming, the University of Colorado Athletic Department, the Denver Broncos, and the Cleveland Indians' minor league teams. She lives in Castle Rock, Colorado with her husband Bruce and her two sons, Matthew and Kevin.

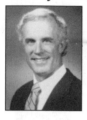

**Harvey S. Newton**, MA, CSCS, is the Director of Program Development for the National Strength and Conditioning Association, and the editor of *Strength & Conditioning*. He served as the 1984 U.S. Olympic Weightlifting Team coach and as national coach from 1981 to 1984. Active in several sports, Newton is the developer of *Strength Training for Cyclists*, a series of videotape strength training instruction videotapes.

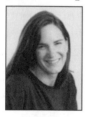

**Julie A. Spotts**, BSEM, is the Product Development Manager at Schwinn Cycling & Fitness, Inc. She has been responsible for the design and production of numerous stationary bikes, recumbent bikes, stair-climbing machines, and various other pieces of fitness equipment, not only at Schwinn, but also for Life Fitness. Her education includes a strong background in bioengineering and biomechanics, and she has conducted research for companies such as AMF Head Racquet Sports and Diversified Products.

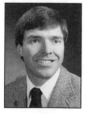

**Wayne L. Westcott**, PhD, is fitness research director at the South Shore YMCA in Quincy, Massachusetts. He is author of several books on strength training and physical fitness, including four editions of the college text, *Strength Fitness*. A former university professor, Wayne has served as a fitness consultant for the YMCA of the USA; the American Council on Exercise; IDEA, the international association of fitness professionals; the President's Council on Physical Fitness and Sports; the International Fitness Institute; and the National Youth Sports Safety Foundation. He has also provided consultation for publications such as *Prevention*, *Men's Health*, *Fitness*, *Club Industry*, *American Fitness Quarterly*, and *Metro Sports*.